MCQs in
Clinical Radiology
Musculoskeletal
Radiology

VOLUME 2

MCQs in Clinical Radiology

Musculoskeletal Radiology

(Question Bank for FRCR)

Prabhakar Rajiah
MBBS MD FRCR
Senior Registrar in Radiology
Manchester
United Kingdom

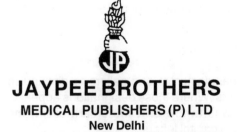

JAYPEE BROTHERS
MEDICAL PUBLISHERS (P) LTD
New Delhi

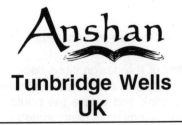

**Tunbridge Wells
UK**

First published in the UK by

Anshan Ltd
in 2006
6 Newlands Road
Tunbridge Wells
Kent TN4 9AT, UK

Tel/Fax: +44 (0)1892 557767
E-mail: info@anshan.co.uk
www.anshan.co.uk

ISBN 1 904798 543

British Library Cataloguing in Publication Data
A catalogue record for this book is available from the British Library

Printed in India by Sanat Printers, Kundli, Haryana

Many of the designations used by manufacturers and sellers to distinguish their products are claimed as trademarks. Where those designations appear in this book and where the publisher was aware of a trademark claim, the designations have been printed in initial capital letters.

Foreword

Radiology is not just X-rays anymore. The rapid strides made in imaging technology has revolutionised radiology with advent of Ultrasound, Computed Tomography, Magnetic Resonance Imaging, PET Scanning and Interventional Radiology. Integration of these recent advances into the syllabus has increased the burden placed on radiology trainees facing Fellowship Exams. There is a burning need for simple and accurate resource to make the process of facing examinations a less daunting task.

In preparing this book, Dr Prabhakar Rajiah has been successful in developing a comprehensive practice resource for the Fellowship Exams. This book is in the same format to the Fellowship exams and has been written using up-to-date and accurate information. This is easily the most extensive and largest collection of MCQs in radiology available today. The main strength of the book the categorisation of questions into related subtopics and the thorough, detailed explanation provided with the answers at the end of each section. The questions are of varying difficulty, covering amongst others, differential diagnosis, epidemiology, which is the staple of any Fellowship Exam and recent imaging techniques. The questions cover the three key components, anatomy, techniques and pathology. This should benefit everyone from the beginner to the more accomplished.

I am in no doubt, that this book is an ideal way of revising for the exams. It is also a good companion for self-assessment and would be of interest for senior radiologists who would like to update their knowledge and stay informed about current practices and imaging methods. This book is an ideal combination of information and revision resource.

Dr Biswaranjan Banerjee MBBS, FRCS, FRCR
Consultant Radiologist
Tameside General Hospital
Manchester
United Kingdom

Preface

Multiple choice questions (MCQs) have now become the standard and the most preferred means of assessing knowledge in all medical specialities including radiology. Along with the tremendous advances made in the various subspecialities of radiology, the level of knowledge not just in depth but also in breadth and the skill required to sit MCQ exams has increased as well. The format of the Fellowship Exams over the recent years has been changed to reflect these advances.

There is no gain saying the fact that the best method of preparing for these exams is keeping abreast of recent advances reading the standard radiology textbooks and journals. However, there is a place for books such as these, which can be used to develop knowledge and hone skills necessary for success in these exams. This book has been written primarily as a revision tool for those sitting MCQ exams in Musculoskeletal Radiology. This book can be approached in two ways. The best way is to read a particular topic in a recognised textbook or journal and subsequently test the knowledge gained using the questions in the corresponding chapter of this book. Alternatively, the book can be used first to identify lacunae in the knowledge base, which can then be corrected using journals and textbooks. It is imperative to realise that while this book cannot be a substitute for textbooks or journals, it can be a valuable revision tool prior to exams. It can also be used by those in an advanced stage, who do not have to stick to any particular format as an informal and fun way of gaining and self-testing radiological knowledge.

The format in this book is the same as used in the Fellowship Exams of the Royal Colleges of UK, Ireland, Hong Kong, Australia and New Zealand. The Royal College of UK Exam has 30 questions to be answered in one and half hours. Each question has five statements with true or false answers. The book has more than 900 questions, each with five statements. Detailed explanations have been provided for the questions at the end of each chapter. The book has been divided into individual chapters, which will enable the reader to assess his strength and weakness, and correct deficiencies in knowledge. Due emphasis has been given to Anatomy, Techniques and Pathology, which are the important components of the Fellowship Exam. A detailed bibliography is provided at the end of this book for further reading.

Prabhakar Rajiah

Contents

Contents

1 Musculoskeletal Imaging

1. **Arthrography:**
   A. Effusion should be aspirated before arthrography
   B. Iohexol is better than ioxaglate
   C. Air introduced for arthrography is absorbed in six hours
   D. Contrast inside a joint will be located close to the needle
   E. Adrenaline hastens the absorption of contrast

2. **Knee arthrography:**
   A. Can be approached only on the medial side of the joint
   B. The site of entry is 2 cm posterior to the patellar mid point
   C. It is vital that the needle enters horizontally to avoid extra-reticular injection
   D. Patient should walk before images are acquired
   E. At least four images are acquired in each quadrant, and valgus strain should be obtained

3. **Wrist arthrography:**
   A. The wrist should be held in horizontally without any degree of flexion
   B. The needle is inserted with an angle of 15 degrees
   C. 4 ml of contrast is optimal
   D. The wrist is usually entered through the volar aspect
   E. Mid point of lower end of ulna is the site for entering wrist joint

4. **Arthrography:**
   A. Ankle is entered by injecting one cm above and medial to the lateral malleolus
   B. Posterior approach gives better images in ankle arthrography
   C. Elbow should be fully extended for arthrography
   D. Elbow is entered between radial head and capitellum
   E. Discomfort in elbow on the second day after examination is abnormal

5. **Indications for hip arthrography:**
   A. Congenital dislocation of hip
   B. Labral tear
   C. Hip prosthesis
   D. Fracture neck of femur
   E. Avascular necrosis

6. **Shoulder arthrography:**
   A. Axial view is required before introducing contrast
   B. The joint is entered one cm below and medial to the coracoid process
   C. The needle should have a slight cranial tilt to avoid injuring glenoid labrum
   D. In delayed images, cartilaginous loose bodies take up the contrast
   E. The arm is internally rotated for proper entry into the joint

7. **Holt-Oram syndrome associated with:**
   A. Hypoplastic thumb
   B. Hypoplastic clavicles
   C. Cardiac septal defects
   D. Co-arctation of aorta
   E. Defect in chest wall

8. **Bilateral symmetrical periosteal reaction in adults seen in:**
   A. Pachydermoperiostotis
   B. Hyperthyroidism
   C. Bronchogenic carcinoma
   D. Fluorosis
   E. Venous insufficiency

9. **Generalized retarded skeletal maturation is seen in:**
   A. Turner's syndrome
   B. Polyostotic fibrous dysplasia
   C. Adrenogenital syndrome
   D. Diabetes mellitus
   E. Congenital heart disease

10. **Accelerated skeletal maturation is seen in:**
    A. Hyperthyroidism
    B. Sotos' syndrome
    C. Rickets
    D. Testicular tumour
    E. Fibrous dysplasia

11. **Hip arthrography:**
    A. If contrast flows away from the needle, it is wrongly placed
    B. 20 ml of contrast injected into prosthesis
    C. Tc colloid injection is more sensitive than contrast media for assessing hip joint
    D. Needle is passed vertically into the femoral neck
    E. For better dissemination of contrast, it has to be exercised

12. **Premature epiphyeal fusion is seen in:**
    A. Down's syndrome
    B. Marfan's syndrome
    C. Haemophilia
    D. Hypothyroidism
    E. Epiphyseal fracture

13. **Erosion of superior aspect of the ribs is seen in:**
    A. Systemic sclerosis
    B. Hyperparathyroidism
    C. Rheumatoid arthritis
    D. SVC obstruction
    E. Poliomyelitis

14. **Acro-osteolysis:**
    A. Syringomyelia
    B. Pemphigus
    C. Neurofibromatosis
    D. Psoriasis
    E. Burns
    F. Pemphigus vulgaris

15. **Acro-osteolysis is seen in:**
    A. Morton's disease
    B. Vinyl chloride poisoning
    C. Progeria
    D. Ehler-Danlos syndrome
    E. Leprosy

16. **Causes of acro-osteolysis:**
    A. Hyperparathyroidism
    B. Insensitivity to pain
    C. Epidermolysis bulloa
    D. Pemphigus vulgaris
    E. Frostbite

17. **Common causes of finger tip calcification:**
    A. Dermatomyositis
    B. Loa loa worm
    C. Guinea worm
    D. SLE
    E. Hyperparathyroidism

18. **Hypertrophic osteoarthropathy-extrathoracic causes:**
    A. Nasopharyngeal carcinoma
    B. Chronic hepatitis
    C. Liver abscess
    D. Gastric ulcer
    E. Amebic dysentery

19. **Associations of syndactyly:**
    A. Carpenter's syndrome
    B. Down's syndrome
    C. Poland's syndrome
    D. Neurofibromatosis
    E. Crozon's syndrome

20. **Associations of brachydactyly:**
    A. Turner's syndrome
    B. Osteomyelitis
    C. Klinefelter's syndrome
    D. Basal cell nevus syndrome
    E. Ellis-van Creveld syndrome

21. **Multicentric epiphyses occurs in:**
    A. Vitamin D toxicity
    B. Cleidocranial dysostosis
    C. Cretinism
    D. NAI
    E. Congenital syphilis

22. **Enlarged thumb is seen in:**
    A. Hyperthyroidism
    B. Hypertrophic pulmonary osteoarthropathy
    C. Neurofibromatosis
    D. Holt-Oram syndrome
    E. Proteus syndrome

23. **Epiphyseal overgrowth is a common feature in:**
    A. Tuberculosis
    B. Eiphyseal dysplasia hemimelica
    C. Healing rickets
    D. Hemophilia
    E. Perthes' disease

24. **Skull defect with sclerosis is seen in:**
    A. Growing fracture   B. Epidermoid cyst
    C. Paget's disease   D. Fibrous dysplasia
    E. Multiple myeloma

25. **Widening of intercondylar notch is seen in:**
    A. Tuberculosis
    B. Gout
    C. Juvenile rheumatoid arthritis
    D. Reiter's disease
    E. Pigmented villonodular synovitis
    F. Osteoarthritis

26. **Widened pubic symphysis is seen in:**
    A. Hyperparathyroidism
    B. Epispadias
    C. Cleidocranial dysplasia
    D. Metastasis
    E. Pregnancy

27. **Widened pubic symphysis is seen in:**
    A. Rheumatoid arthritis
    B. Prune-belly syndrome
    C. Ankylosing spondylitis
    D. Gout
    E. Prostate metastasis

28. **Multiple ossification centers in the epiphysis are seen in:**
    A. Syphilis
    B. Cleidocranial dysplasia
    C. Down's syndrome
    D. Scurvy
    E. Cretinism

29. **Permeative pattern in mid shaft of 15-year-old:**
    A. Histiocytosis
    B. Osteomyelitis
    C. Neuroblastoma
    D. Osteosarcoma
    E. Ewing's sarcoma

30. **Plantar calcaneal spur is seen in:**
    A. Osteoarthritis   B. Rheumatoid arthritis
    C. Ankylosing spondylitis D. DISH
    E. Reiter's disease

31. **Epiphyseolysis is seen in:**
    A. Renal osteodystrophy
    B. Hypothyroidism
    C. Radiation
    D. Steroids
    E. SUFE

32. **Short ribs are seen in:**
    A. Achondroplasia
    B. Ellis-van Creveld syndrome
    C. Jeune's syndrome
    D. Majewski syndrome
    E. Ollier's disease

33. **Calcified loose bodies in joint seen in:**
    A. Synovial cell sarcoma
    B. Synovial osteochondromatosis
    C. Osteochondritis dissecans
    D. Charcots joints
    E. Tuberculosis

34. **Terminal phalangeal sclerosis seen in:**
    A. Rheumatoid arthritis
    B. Scleroderma
    C. Osteoid osteoma
    D. SLE
    E. Sarcoidosis

35. **Periosteal reaction is seen in:**
    A. Fibrous dysplasia
    B. Thalassemia
    C. Juvenile rheumatoid arthritis
    D. Sarcoidosis
    E. Reiter's disease

36. **Endosteal scalloping is seen in:**
    A. Gaucher's disease
    B. Myeloma
    C. Leukemia
    D. Lymphoma
    E. Chondrosarcoma

37. **Erosion at the outer end of the clavicle:**
    A. Paget's disease   B. Post traumatic
    C. CA breast   D. Hyperparathyroidism
    E. RA

38. **Causes of clinodactyly:**
    A. Down's syndrome
    B. Morquio's syndrome
    C. Hurler's syndrome
    D. Arthritis
    E. Trauma

39. **Associations of polydactyly:**
    A. Trisomy 13
    B. Carpenter's syndrome
    C. Ellis-von Creveld syndrome
    D. Marfans syndrome
    E. Madelung's syndrome

40. **Ribbon ribs are seen in:**
    A. Neurofibromatosis
    B. Marfan's syndrome
    C. Rheumatoid arthritis
    D. Osteogenesis imperfecta
    E. Fibrous dysplasia

41. **The following are causes of dense ribs:**
    A. Sickle cell anemia
    B. Mastocytosis
    C. Osteopetrosis
    D. Metastases
    E. Fluorosis

42. **Widening of ribs seen in:**
    A. Paget's disease
    B. Hurler's disease
    C. Thalassemia
    D. Fibrous dysplasia
    E. Rickets

43. **Bulbous enlargment of costochondral junction:**
    A. Neurofibromatosis
    B. Down's syndrome
    C. Rickets
    D. Achondroplasia
    E. Scurvy

44. **Expansile lesion in the rib is seen in:**
    A. Tuberculosis   B. Enchondrome
    C. ABC   D. Plasmacytoma
    E. Eosinophilic granuloma

45. **Superior notching of ribs is seen in:**
    A. Neurofibromatosis
    B. Marfan's syndrome
    C. Restrictive lung disease
    D. SLE
    E. Scleroderma

46. **Inferior notching of ribs:**
    A. Neurofibromatosis
    B. Thalassemia
    C. Hyperparathyroidism
    D. Tetralogy of Fallot
    E. Poliomyelitis

47. **Causes of pencilled distal end of clavicle:**
    A. Progeria
    B. Scleroderma
    C. Hypoparathyroidism
    D. Eosinophilic granuloma
    E. Cleidocranial dysplasia

48. **Intraorbital calcification is seen in:**
    A. Drusen
    B. Retinoblastoma
    C. Vitreous hemorrhage
    D. Pseudotumour
    E. Lymphoma

49. **Sunburst periosteal reaction is seen in:**
    A. Tropical ulcer
    B. Meningioma
    C. Tuberous sclerosis
    D. Caffey's disease
    E. DISH

50. **Common causes of erosion of medial end of the clavicle:**
    A. Eosinophilic granuloma
    B. Lymphoma
    C. Sarcoma
    D. Metastases
    E. Tuberculosis

51. **Leontiasis ossea:**
    A. Paget's disease
    B. Fibrous dysplasia
    C. Neurofibromatosis
    D. Marfan's disease
    E. Leprosy

52. **Fragmented epiphysis is seen in:**
    A. Rickets   B. Mucopolysaccharidosis
    C. Cretinism   D. Epiphyseal dysplasia
    E. Schmidts dysplasia

53. **Short 4th metacarpal is seen in:**
    A. Turner's syndrome
    B. Klinefelter's syndrome
    C. Down's syndrome
    D. Diaphyseal aclasia
    E. Melorheostosis

54. **Excessive callus formation is seen in:**
    A. Acromegaly
    B. Paget's disease
    C. Osteopetrosis
    D. Osteogenesis imperfecta
    E. Neuropathic arthropathy

55. **Delayed eruption of teeth seen in:**
    A. Myxedema
    B. Osteogenesis imperfecta
    C. Cleidocranial dysostosis
    D. Hypophosphatasia
    E. Hyperparathyroidism

56. **Common causes of sausage digit:**
    A. Tuberculous dactylitis is the most common cause
    B. Psoriasis
    C. Osteomyelitis
    D. Thalassemia
    E. Sarcoidosis

57. **Onion skin periosteal reaction is seen in:**
    A. Osteosarcoma
    B. Ewing's sarcoma
    C. Eosinophilic granuloma
    D. Leukemia
    E. Osteomyelitis

58. **Localised enlargement of bone is seen in:**
    A. Diaphyseal aclasia
    B. Homocystinuria
    C. Gaucher's disease
    D. Neurofibromatosis
    E. Haemophilia

59. **Differential diagnosis of flat femoral capital epiphysis:**
    A. Cretinism
    B. Sarcoidosis
    C. Multiple epiphyseal dysplasia
    D. Osteoporosis
    E. Cushing's syndrome

60. **Ring epiphysis is seen in:**
    A. Osteoporosis   B. Rickets
    C. Hypothyroidism   D. Juvenile rheumatoid
    E. Scurvy

61. **Hyperlucent ribs are seen in:**
    A. Rickets   B. Scurvy
    C. Osteopetrosis   D. Acromegaly
    E. Cushing's

62. **Causes of increased carpal angle:**
    A. Down's syndrome   B. Arthrogryposis
    C. Hurler's syndrome   D. Morquio's syndrome
    E. Madelung's deformity

63. **Lumbar spine X-ray:**
    A. Radiation dose is 40 times that of chest X-ray
    B. There is good correlation between degenerative changes in X-ray and severity of back pain
    C. Two thirds of elderly population. >55 years, have degenerative changes
    D. 10% incidence of tumours in those with back pain
    E. Very sensitive for detection of tumours and infections

64. **Common causes of erosion of medial end of the clavicle:**
    A. Eosinophilic granuloma
    B. Lymphoma
    C. Sarcoma
    D. Metastases
    E. Tuberculosis

65. **Ulnar deviation in the absence of erosions:**
    A. Osteoarthritis
    B. SLE
    C. Jaccoud's arthropathy
    D. Psoriasis
    E. Rheumatoid arthritis

66. **Following statements are true:**
    A. In recurrent dislocation of the patella, medial displacement is characteristic
    B. Stress fractures of the foot are most commonly seen in the fifth metatarsal
    C. Avascular necrosis is a complication of fracture of the talar neck
    D. Fractures of the base of the fifth metatarsal usually follow inversion injuries
    E. Presence of gas in the painful shoulder suggests septic arthritis

67. **Pseudoarthrosis is seen in:**
    A. Osteogenesis imperfecta
    B. Neurofibromatosis
    C. Fibrous dysplasis
    D. Paget's disease
    E. Ankylosing spondylitis

68. **Heel pad thickening is seen in:**
    A. Obesity
    B. Myxedema
    C. Epileptics
    D. Rheumatoid arthritis
    E. Hyperparathyroidism

69. **Causes of pain in those with hip prosthesis:**
    A. Trochanteric bursitis
    B. Fracture of prosthesis
    C. Dislocation
    D. Heterotopic ossification
    E. Sarcoma

70. **Causes of marginal erosions:**
    A. Rheumatoid arthritis
    B. CPPD
    C. Ankylosing spondylitis
    D. Pigmented villonodular synovitis
    E. Gout

71. **Associations of club foot:**
    A. Neurofibromatosis
    B. Spina bifida
    C. Arthrogryposis multiplex congenita
    D. Myelomeningocele
    E. Chondrodysplasia punctata

ANSWERS

1. **A-T, B-F, C-F, D-F, E-F**
   If effusion is not aspirated, the contrast will be diluted. Ioxaglate is better than iohexol, since it is absorbed slowly. Contrast is absorbed in few hours, but air takes four days. Contrast will spread freely within the confines of the joint. Adrenaline delays the absorption of contrast and hence used, if a long examination is expected.

2. **A-F, B-T, C-F, D-T, E-T**
   Knee joint can be approached either from the medial or the lateral side. The site of entry is 1-2 cm behind the mid point of patella. The needle is directed anteriorly to avoid infrapatellar pad of fat. Valgus or varus strain is necessary for obtaining good images.

3. **A-F, B-F, C-T, D-F, E-F**
   The wrist is held with 10 degrees of flexion. The needle is inserted with 15 degrees angulation. The wrist is entered through the dorsal aspect of the midpoint of distal end of radius.

4. **A-F, B-F, C-F, D-T, E-F**
   Ankle is entered anteriorly, 1 cm above and lateral to medial malleolus. Elbow should be flexed for proper injection. Discomfort is common in any joint for two days after arthrography.

5. **A-T, B-T, C-T, D-F, E-T**
   Loose bodies and proximal femoral deficiency are other well known indication.

6. **A-T, B-F, C-F, D-T, E-F**
   AP views in internal and external rotation are also required. Joint is entered one cm below and lateral to the cricoid process. The arms are kept supinated by the side of the body and they are not internally rotated. Needle is inserted vertically downwards.

7. **A-T, B-T, C-T, D-T, E-F**
   Holt-Oram syndrome (Heart Hand syndrome); AD (Chromosome 12)
   ASD (secundum)/VSD (muscular)/Conduction defects/other anomalies, Aplasia/hypoplasia/fusion of radius/carpal/thenar bones Phocomelia can be seen Sprengel shoulder/clavicle abnormalities coarctation/aortic arch anomalies are seen rarely.

8. **A-T, B-F, C-T, D-T, E-T**
   Seen in hypothyroidism not hyperthyroidism. Bronchogenic carcinoma produces hypertrophic pulmonary osteoarthropathy, which produces bilateral symmetrical periosteal reaction and soft tissue swelling. Chronic venous insufficiency is a known cause of periosteal reaction. Hypervitaminosis A is another cause.

9. **A-T, B-F, C-F, D-T, E-T**
   Chronic diseases—Heart disease, respiratory(cystic fibrosis and other chronic diseases) renal, inflammatory bowel disease, malnutrition, rickets
   Endocrine—Hypopituitarism, hypothyroidism, hypogonadism, Cushing's, Genetic-Trisomy 18, 21
   Bony dysplasias

10. **A-T, B-T, C-F, D-T, E-T**
    Idiopathic, Hormonal—hypothalamic, adrenal, gonadal tumours, hyperthyroidism, pseudohypoparathyroidism, McCune Albright syndrome, Sotos' syndrome, Weaver Smith syndrome,Marshall Smith syndrome

11. **A-F, B-T, C-T, D-T, E-T**
    Normally, upto 5 ml of contrast is injected. More is injected if there is a prosthesis.

12. **A-F, B-F, C-T, D-F, E-T**
    Radiation, burns, sickle cell anemia, infarcts, Ollier's disease.

13. **A-T, B-T, C-T, D-F, E-T**
    SLE, Sjögren's, Neurofibromatosis, OI, Marfan's, lung disease.

14. **A-T, B-F, C-T, D-T, E-T, F-F**

15. **A-T, B-T, C-T, D-T, E-T**

16. **A-T, B-T, C-T, D-F, E-T**
    Hyperparathyroidism, vinyl chloride poisoning, frostbite, epidermolysis bullosa, insensitivity to pain, Morton's disease, leprosy,diabetes, Reiter's syndrome, progeria, pyknodysostosis, TAO, Raynaud's disease, dermatomyositis, Ehlers-Danlos syndrome atherosclerosis are other causes.

17. **A-T, B-F, C-F, D-T, E-T**
    Scleroderma, CREST syndrome, dermatomyositis, hyperparathyroidism, SLE, Raynaud's are causes of finger tip calcification.

18. **A-T, B-T, C-T, D-T, E-T**
    Other causes are ulcerative colitis, Crohn's disease, lymphoma, gastric carcinoma, cirrhosis, cholangiocarcinoma, pancreatic carcinoma, CML are other causes.

19. **A-T, B-T, C-T, D-T, E-F**
    Crouzon's syndrome is craniosynostosis

20. **A-T, B-T, C-F, D-T, E-T**
    Brachydactyly is shortening of digits.
    Trauma, arthritis, dysplasias, pseudohypoparathyroidism, pseudopseudohypoparathyroidism are other causes.

21. **A-F, B-F, C-T, D-T, E-T**

22. **A-F, B-T, C-T, D-F, E-F**
Klipple-Trenaunay syndrome, hemangiomas, Maffucci's syndrome, macrodystrophia lipomatosa are other causes.

23. **A-T, B-T, C-F, D-T, E-T**
Hemophilia and JRA are common causes.
Pyogenic, fungal arthritis and fibrous dysplasia are other causes.

24. **A-F, B-F, C-F, D-T, E-F**
Epidermoid cyst, meningocele, hemangioma, histiocytosis, chronic osteomyelitis, fibrous dysplasia and frontal sinus mucocele are the common causes of lytic lesion with sclerosis.

25. **A-T, B-T, C-T, D-F, E-T, F-F**
Widening of intercondylar notch is seen in haemophilia, juvenile rheumatoid arthritis, rheumatoid arthritis, gout, pigmented villonodular synovitis, psoriasis and tuberculosis.

26. **A-T, B-T, C-T, D-T, E-T**

27. **A-T, B-T, C-T, D-F, E-F**
10 mm in newborn and > 8 mm in adults. Pregnancy, trauma, osteitis pubis, osteomyelitis, lytic metastasis, hyperparathyroidism, ankylosing spondylitis, rheumatoid arthritis, congenital conditions-ectopia vesicae, epispadias, hypospadias, prune-belly syndrome, cleidocranial dysplasia.

28. **A-F, B-F, C-T, D-F, E-T**
Morquio's syndrome avascular necrosis, chondrodysplasia punctate, trisomy 18, fetal warfarin syndrome, fetal alcohol syndrome are othe causes.

29. **A-T, B-T, C-T, D-T, E-T**
Other causes are leukemia and lymphoma. Early stage of histiocytosis shows a permeative pattern with wide transition margin and laminated periosteal reaction.

30. **A-T, B-T C-T, D-T, E-T**
Plantar calcaneal spur is common in seronegative arthropathies like ankylosing spondylitis, psoriasis, Reiter's disease. It is occasionally seen in rheumatoid arthritis, osteoarthritis and diffuse idiopathic skeletal hyperostosis.

31. **A-T, B-T, C-T, D-T, E-T**

32. **A-T, B-T, C-T, D-T, E-T**

33. **A-F, B-T, C-T, D-T, E-F**
Calcified loose bodies inside joints are seen in Osteochondritis dissecans, osteochondral fractures, detached osteophytes, Charcots joints and synovial osteochondromatosis.

34. **A-T, B-T, C-F, D-T, E-T**
    Scleroderma, sarcoid, SLE and rheumatoid arthritis are the causes of terminal phalangeal sclerosis.

35. **A-F, B-F, C-T, D-T, E-T**

36. **A-T, B-T, C-T, D-T, E-T**
    Fibrous dysplasia, eosinophilic granuloma, enchondroma are other causes.

37. **A-T, B-T, C-T, D-T, E-T**
    Rheumatoid arthritis, hyperparathyroidism, metastasis, myeloma, trauma, cleidocranial dysostosis.

38. **A-T, B-F, C-F, D-T, E-T**
    Clinodactyly is curvature of finger. Down's syndrome, tauma, arthritis and contractures are causes of clinodactyly.

39. **A-T, B-T, C-T, D-F, E-F**
    Laurence-Moon-Biedel syndrome, Meckel-Gruber syndrome.

40. **A-T, B-F, C-T, D-T, E-F**
    Resection, hyperparathyroidism, Morquio's, polymyositis, scleroderma, juvenile idiopathic arthritis, severe osteoporosis are other causes.

41. **A-T, B-T, C-T, D-T, E-T**
    Pyknodysostosis and other sclerosing dysplasias.

42. **A-T, B-T, C-T, D-T, E-F**
    Achondroplasia another cause. Healed fracture with callus is a cause.

43. **A-F, B-F, C-T, D-T, E-T**
    Jeune's syndrome, fibrous dysplasia are other causes.

44. **A-T, B-T, C-T, D-T, E-T**
    Fibrous dysplasia, Ewing's, lymphoma are other causes.

45. **A-T, B-T, C-T, D-T, E-T**
    RA, hyperparathyroidism are other causes.

46. **A-T, B-T, C-T, D-T, E-T**
    Coarctation is the most common cause. Other causes are occlusion of aorta or subclavian artery, including thrombosis, embolism, absent pulmonary artery, pulmonary stenosis, Taussig Blalock shunt, SVC obstruction, AV malformation of systemic or pulmonary arteries.

47. **A-T, B-T, C-F, D-F, E-F**
    Hyperparathyroidism, infection are other causes.

48. **A-T, B-T, C-T, D-F, E-F**
Retinoblastoma is the most common cause of calcification in children.

49. **A-T, B-T, C-F, D-F, E-F**
Osteosarcoma is the most common cause of a sunburst type of periosteal reaction. It is not specific for osteosarcoma and is also seen in osteomyelitis. Ewing's sarcoma and other tumours can occasionally show this pattern of periosteal reaction.

50. **A-T, B-T, C-T, D-T, E-T**
Erosion of the medial end of clavicle is less common than the lateral end of clavicle.

51. **A-T, B-T, C-F, D-F, E-F**
Leontiasis ossea is lion like face due to overgrowth of facial bones. Thick bones with obliteration of sinuses seen. Also seen in cranio metaphyseal dysplasia.

52. **A-F, B-F, C-T, D-T, E-F**
Down's, Morquio's, chondrodysplasia punctate are other causes

53. **A-T, B-T, C-F, D-T, E-T**
Pseudohypoparathyroidism, pseudo-pseudohypoparathyroidism, basal cell nevus syndrome, Cornelia de Lange's syndrome are other causes.
This is measured by drawing a tangent between 4th and 5th metatarsal. Normally it should pass above the head of 3rd metatarsal. If it intersects the third metatarsal, it is due to shortening of fourth metatarsal.

54. **A-F, B-F, C-F, D-T, E-T**
Steroids, congenital insensitivity to pain, paralysis, renal osteodystrophy, battered child and multiple myeloma are other causes.

55. **A-T, B-T, C-T, D-T, E-F**
Congenital hypothyroidism, Down's syndrome, osteopetrosis, Gaucher's disease, radiotherapy, frontometaphyseal dysplasias, Cornelia de Lange's syndrome are other causes.

56. **A-F, B-T, C-T, D-F, E-T**
Sausage digit refers to fusiform swelling of the digits. The most common cause is psoriasis. Other causes are sarcoidosis, osteomyelitis, tuberculosis and sickle cell disease.

57. **A-T, B-T, C-F, D-F, E-T**

58. **A-T, B-F, C-T, D-T, E-T**
Hyperemia, NF, Proteus syndrome, Klippel-Trenaunay syndrome.

59. **A-T, B-F, C-T, D-T, E-T**
    Steroids, osteogenesis imperfecta, NAI, neuropathic arthropathy, renal osteodystrophy, myeloma. Steroid use and Cushing's syndrome produce avascular necrosis which flattens and deforms the femoral head with preservation of the joint space.

60. **A-T, B-T, C-F, D-F, E-T**

61. **A-F, B-T, C-T, D-T, E-T**

62. **A-F, B-F, C-T, D-T, E-T**
    Carpal angle is formed between tangents to proximal row of carpal bones. It is normally 130 degrees. Increased in Madelung's, Turner's, Hurler's and Morquio's syndrome.
    Decreased in Down's syndrome, arthrogryposis, bone dysplasia.

63. **A-T, B-F, C-T, D-F, E-F**
    Lumbar spine X-ray is not sensitive for diagnosis of tumours and infections and is not of much use in degenerative changes. A routine lumbar spine X-ray for back pain is not preferred. Less than 1% have back pain.

64. **A-T, B-T, C-T, D-T, E-T**
    Erosion of the medial end of clavicle is less common than the lateral end of clavicle.

65. **A-F, B-T, C-T, D-F, E-F**

66. **A-F, B-T, C-T, D-T, E-F**
    In patellar dislocation, lateral displacement is characteristic. Presence of gas in joints could be a normal process, such as osteoarthritis.

67. **A-T, B-T, C-T, D-F, E-T**
    Causes of pseudoarthrosis are: Non-union of fracture, congenital, osteogenesis imperfecta, neurofibromatosis, cleidocranial dysplasia, fibrous dysplasia and ankylosing spondylitis.

68. **A-T, B-T, C-T, D-F, E-F**
    Heel pad is thickened in males if it measures more than 23 mm and in females if more than 21.5 mm. The causes are acromegaly, myxedema, phenytoin toxicity, obesity, infection and oedema.

69. **A-T, B-T, C-T, D-T, E-F**

70. **A-T, B-F, C-T, D-T, E-T**
    Marginal erosions are intra-articular erosions that occur in portions of bone that are not covered by articular cartilage. The most common cause is rheumatoid arthritis.

71. **A-T, B-T, C-T, D-T, E-T**

2 *Arthropathies*

1. **Causes of subchondral cystic lesions:**
   - A. Benign fibrous histiocytoma
   - B. Pigmented villonodular synovitis
   - C. Giant cell tumour
   - D. Ganglion
   - E. Hemophilia

2. **Pigmented villonodular synovitis (PVNS):**
   - A. More common in women
   - B. Metacarpal joint is the most common joint involved
   - C. Seen in older age group
   - D. Calcification is common in the soft tissue lesion
   - E. Subarticular erosions are characteristic

3. **PVNS:**
   - A. Erosions are more common in hip than in the knee
   - B. Periarticular osteoporosis is a common feature
   - C. Earliest change is joint space narrowing
   - D. Soft tissue is dense
   - E. Scalloping of fat pad in MRI

4. **PVNS:**
   - A. Pigment is always seen in pathological specimens
   - B. Can be completely extracapsular
   - C. Angiography shows AV malformation
   - D. Soft tissue nodules calcify
   - E. Erosions are more common in tight joints

5. **MRI shows intra-articular hemosiderin in the following conditions:**
   - A. Neuropathic joints
   - B. Synovial osteochondromatosis
   - C. Synovial hemangioma
   - D. Synovial sarcoma
   - E. Hemophilia

6. **Features of homocystinuria:**
   A. Premature degeneration of articular cartilage
   B. Renal calculi
   C. Kyphoscoliosis
   D. Loosers zones
   E. Increased metacarpal index

7. **Features of juvenile chronic arthritis:**
   A. Periosteal reaction
   B. Pulmonary fibrosis
   C. Bony ankylosis
   D. Amyloid deposition
   E. Narrowing of metacarpals

8. **Ankylosis of interphalangeal joints:**
   A. Reiter's
   B. Still's disease
   C. Ankylosing spondylitis
   D. Erosive osteoarthritis
   E. Gout

9. **Common causes of arthritis of interphalangeal joints of great toe:**
   A. Degeneration
   B. Rheumatoid
   C. Reiter's
   D. Gout
   E. SLE

10. **Fusion of sacroiliac joint is seen in:**
    A. Tuberculosis
    B. Metastasis
    C. Reactive arthritis
    D. Reiter's
    E. Psoriasis

11. **Synovial disease with decreased signal intensity in MRI:**
    A. Pigmented villonodular synovitis
    B. Synovial haematoma
    C. Synovial hemangioma
    D. Hemophilia
    E. Rheumatoid arthritis

12. **Decreased periarticular bone density is seen in:**
    A. Gout   B. Psoriasis
    C. Rheumatoid   D. Haemophilia
    E. Tuberculosis

13. **Features of epidermolysis bullosa:**
    A. Soft tissue webbing between digits
    B. Cystic changes in lungs
    C. Proximal esophageal stricture
    D. Amputation of phalanges
    E. Soft tissue dystrophic calcification

14. **Soft tissue ossification:**
    A. Burn's
    B. Stress fractures
    C. Parosteal osteosarcoma
    D. Paraplegia
    E. Osteogenesis imperfecta

15. **Carpal fusion:**
    A. Scapholunoid fusion is the most common
    B. Most commonly occurs in the same carpal row
    C. Occurs in arthrogryposis multiplex congenita
    D. Is syndrome related if it affects both the rows
    E. Seen in Madelung's deformity

16. **Ankylosing spondylitis:**
    A. Pseudoarthrosis is called Anderson's lesions
    B. Carrot stick fracture is fracture through an ankylosed segment
    C. Romanus lesion is erosion at site of insertion of annulus fibrosis
    D. Squaring of vertebral bodies is due to periostitis
    E. Sydesmophytes are inflammatory ossification of spinal ligaments

17. **Common causes of carpal fusion:**
    A. Aperts syndrome
    B. Still's disease
    C. Homocystinuria
    D. Holt-Oram's syndrome
    E. Chondroectodermal dysplasia

18. **Ankylosing spondylitis is associated with:**
    A. Mitral regurgitation   B. Basal fibrosis
    C. Amyloidosis   D. Iritis
    E. Heart block

19. **Ankylosing spondylitis:**
    A. MCP joints are more commonly affected than the hip joints
    B. C 1/2 subluxation occurs
    C. HLA B 27 is seen in more than 80%
    D. SI joints are less often affected in females
    E. Increased incidence of psoriasis in close relatives

20. **Ankylosing spondylitis:**
    A. Restriction of expansion of chest is commonly due to upper zone fibrosis
    B. Peripheral joints are involved in 50% of cases
    C. Sciatica can be seen bilaterally or alternate from side-to-side
    D. The articular surface of sacroiliac joint can be visualized through the ankylosed joint
    E. Dagger sign is due to ossification of paraspinal ligaments

21. **Ankylosing spondylitis:**
    A. The synovitis in ankylosing spondylitis is less than that of rheumatoid arthritis
    B. There is no formation of lamellar bone in the enthesophytes
    C. Heart block is a well known complication
    D. Chronic prostatitis is a recognized complication
    E. Iritis is seen in 25% of individuals

22. **Ankylosing spondylitis:**
    A. The density of odontoid process is increased
    B. Vertebral bodies are osteoporotic
    C. Hatchet erosions are seen on the medial aspect of head of humerus
    D. Changes in peripheral joints are bilaterally symmetrical
    E. No periarticular osteoporos is unlike rheumatoid

23. **Ankylosing spondylitis:**
    A. Affects and causes ankylosis of joint prosthesis
    B. Arachnoid diverticulum is a characteristic feature
    C. Trochanters are not usually affected by the enthesopathy
    D. Rotator cuff tear can occur
    E. Resorption of distal end of clavicle is a late complication

24. **Premature osteoarthritis is common in:**
    A. Charcot's   B. Acromegaly
    C. Ochronosis   D. Epiphyseal dysplasia
    E. Pigmented villonodular synovitis

25. **Spondylolisthesis:**
    A. There is increased incidence of spina bifida occulta in spondylolisthesis
    B. There is high prevalence of spondylolysis in Eskimos
    C. Inverted Napoleans hat sign is very specific for L4/5 spondylolisthesis
    D. The spinous process of the vertebra is rotated
    E. Pars defect is best visualized in AP angulated view with cephalad tilt of 30°

26. **Recognised causes of spondylolisthesis:**
    A. Increased lumbar lordosis
    B. Metastasis at parts interarticularis
    C. Weakness of ligaments
    D. Birth fracture
    E. Separate ossification centers of pars interarticularis

27. **Spondylolisthesis:**
    A. In true spondylolisthesis, a step off is seen above the level of slip
    B. The angle between long axis of pedicle and long axis of articular pillar is increased in degerative spondylolisthesis
    C. Thick bony buttress extends from the sacral promontory
    D. Stepladder sign is seen if a line through the plane of each apophyseal joint passes through the space below its level or lies anterior to it
    E. The spinous process of the affected vertebra is felt prominent in the back, in spondylolysis

28. **Causes of unilateral spondylolisthesis:**
    A. Spina bifida   B. Bone island
    C. Osteoid osteoma   D. Paget's disease
    E. Sarcoidosis

29. **Gout:**
    A. Usually starts before 20 years
    B. Associated with nephrocalcinosis
    C. Increased incidence in patients with lymphoma
    D. Tophi commonly calcify
    E. Most commonly affects 1st MTPJ

30. **Gout:**
    A. Causes erosions extending beyond the articular margins
    B. Cause increased heel pad thickness
    C. Cause widened intercondylar notch
    D. Joint space loss is very late
    E. Does not cause cord compression

31. **Gout:**
    A. The latent period between first clinical symptom and X-ray abnormality is atleast five years
    B. Soft tissue swelling is the earliest finding
    C. Tophi will be deposited only in vascular areas
    D. Shelf like elevated bony margin is a salient finding
    E. The erosions are not seen within the joint

32. **Subtypes of synovial joints:**
    A. Proximal radioulnar—pivot joint
    B. Knee joint—hinge joint
    C. First carpometacarpal joint—plane joint
    D. Temporomandibular—bicondylar joint
    E. Shoulder joint—spheroidal joint

33. **Amniotic bands:**
    A. Caused by premature rupture of chorion
    B. Most common in the first pregnancy
    C. Associated with club feet
    D. Bilaterally symmetrical
    E. Constrictions are seen in the soft tissue and bone is spared

34. **Differential diagnosis for multiple cyst like lesions of metacarpals and phalanges:**
    A. Fibrous dysplasia
    B. Sarcoidosis
    C. Tuberous sclerosis
    D. Vinyl chloride
    E. Epidermolysis bullosa

35. **Common features of musculoskeletal sarcoidosis:**
    A. Nasal bone destruction is characteristic
    B. Sclerosis of terminal phalanges
    C. Acro-osteolysis
    D. Paraspinal soft tissue
    E. Acute polyarthritis

36. **The following are complications of steroids:**
    A. Soft tissue atrophy
    B. Neuropathic joints
    C. Rupture of tendons
    D. Septic arthritis
    E. Carpal tunnel syndrome

37. **Causes of H shaped vertebrae:**
    A. Sickle cell disease
    B. Thalassemia
    C. Heriditary spherocytosis
    D. Gaucher's disease
    E. Paget's disease

38. **Causes of cupids bow shaped vertebra:**
    A. Osteoporosis   B. Sickle cell disease
    C. Osteomalacia   D. Normal variant
    E. Paget's disease

39. **Common causes of fish shaped vertebrae:**
    A. Normal appearance   B. Paget's disease
    C. Osteoporosis   D. Sickle cell disease
    E. Osteomalacia

40. **Osteoporosis:**
    A. The indentation caused by osteoporosis is irregular, but that of osteomalacia is smooth
    B. Compression fracture does not involve the middle column of the spine
    C. In osteoporosis, compression fractures are seen, but burst fractures are rare
    D. All burst fractures in osteoporosis are unstable
    E. Any fracture above level of C7, in osteoporosis, is due to second pathology

41. **Features of alkaptonuria:**
    A. All cases of alkaptonuria progress to arthropathy
    B. Earliest spinal changes are seen in the sacroiliac joint
    C. The outer fibers of annulus are typically affected
    D. Cervical spine is the most common part to be involved in discal calcification
    E. There is no intervertebral space narrowing even in advanced cases

42. **Untreated SLE can result in:**
    A. Avascular necrosis of the femoral head
    B. Erosions around the joints
    C. General osteoporosis
    D. Periosteal new bone formation
    E. Pericarditis

43. **Sarcoidosis:**
    A. Very frequently seen without skin or pulmonary involvement
    B. Periosteal reaction is a common feature
    C. Punched out appearance is a typical feature of sarcoidosis
    D. Spine is the most common site involved in musculoskeletal sarcoidosis
    E. Proximal phalanges are the most common part of hand to be involved

44. **Differential diagnosis of arthritis with normal bone density:**
    A. PVNS   B. Gout
    C. Psoriasis   D. Hemophilia
    E. Scleroderma

45. **Calcification of articular cartilage occurs in:**
    A. Hemochromatosis   B. Ochronosis
    C. Osteoarthritis   D. Hyperparathyroidism
    E. Rheumatoid

46. **Hemochromatosis:**
    A. MCP joints are characteristically affected
    B. May result in cardiomyopathy
    C. Basal ganglia may be calcified
    D. High density in bone
    E. Carpometacarpal joints spared

47. **Hypertorphic osteoarthropathy:**
    A. Malignant mesothelioma is a recognized cause
    B. Most common etiology is small cell carcinoma of bronchus
    C. Pain is relieved by vagotomy distal to the origin of the recurrent laryngeal nerve
    D. Symmetrical arthropathy is the hallmark
    E. There is associated soft tissue swelling of periarticular region

48. **Hypertrophic pulmonary osteoarthropathy is seen in:**
    A. Lung abscess   B. Leiomyoma esophagus
    C. Thymoma   D. Lung cyst
    E. Interstitial fibrosis of lung

49. **Hypertrophic pulmonary osteoarthropathy:**
    A. Bone scan shows periarticular uptake
    B. Diffuse bilateral uptake is characteristic
    C. Epiphysis is spared
    D. Mandible is abnormal in 40% of bone scans
    E. Scapula is involved in 2/3rd of cases

50. **Hypertrophic pulmonary osteoarthropathy:**
    A. Periosteal reaction disappears after thoracotomy
    B. Distal phalanges are not affected
    C. Affects the dorsal and medial aspect of long bone
    D. The periosteal reaction is rough throughout the course of disease
    E. Clubbing is associated
    F. Epiphysis involved only in cyanotic heart disease

51. **Jaccoud's arthropathy:**
    A. Seen in rheumatic heart disease
    B. Juxta-articular ostepenia
    C. Erosions are not seen
    D. Joint space narrowing
    E. Flexion of MCP marked in 4th and 5th Finger

52. **Rheumatoid arthritis:**
    A. Pleural effusions are more common in women
    B. Manubriosternal joint may be affected
    C. Amyloidosis is recognized sequelae
    D. 15% have splenomegaly
    E. Keratoconjunctivitis can occur
    F. Severity of lung disease related to severity of arthritis

53. **Rheumatoid arthritis:**
    A. Soft tissue swelling during acute attacks
    B. Soft tissue medial to ulnar styloid is an early sign
    C. Affects upper limb more than lower limb
    D. Cystic expansion of carpal bones may occur
    E. Carpal fusion is a recognized complication

54. **Associations of rheumatoid arthritis:**
    A. Encephalitis   B. Myopathy
    C. Empyema   D. Glomerulonephritis
    E. Swan neck deformity uncommon

55. **Radiological changes of rheumatoid:**
    A. Erosion of pisiform
    B. Erosion of non-articulating surface of ulnar styloid
    C. Erosion of intervertebral end plate is very uncommon
    D. Odontoid erosion
    E. Cervicodorsal junction most common area involved in spine

56. **Protrusio acetabuli is seen in:**
    A. Reiter's syndrome   B. Osteogenesis imperfecta
    C. Ankylosing spondylitis D. Cushing's
    E. Marfan's syndrome

57. **Sacroiliitis is seen in:**
    A. Ankylosing spondylitis
    B. Osteitis condensans ilii
    C. Rheumatoid arthritis
    D. Acromegaly
    E. Infection

58. **The following conditions produce bilaterally symmetrical sacroiliitis:**
    A. Enteropathic   B. Psoriasis
    C. Reiter's   D. Rheumatoid
    E. Ochronosis

59. **Scleroderma:**
    A. Bronchogenic carcinoma is associated
    B. Proximal interphalangeal joint is the commonly affected
    C. Raynaud's phenomenon is a common presenting feature
    D. 10% have rheumatoid type erosive arthropathy
    E. Increased incidence of carcinoma esophagus

60. **Reiter's disease:**
    A. Major joints are commonly involved
    B. Females are commonly affected
    C. Orogenital ulceration occurs in more than 50% of patients
    D. Can present as arthropathy of interphalangeal joints of feet
    E. Does not affect large joints of upper limb

61. **Reiter's syndrome:**
    A. Causes paravertebral ossification
    B. Periosteal reaction is commonly seen
    C. Causes enthesopathy
    D. Osteoporosis in chronic disease
    E. Limb involvement bilaterally symmetrical

62. **Rheumatoid arthritis:**
    A. Terry Thomas sign is separation of lunate and pisiform
    B. Zig zag deformity is ulnar deviation and carpal radial rotation
    C. The cervical spinous processes are tapered
    D. In discal involvement there is loss of disc height and end plate sclerosis
    E. Produces shortening of neck length

63. **Rheumatoid arthritis:**
    A. Mallet finger—persistent extension of DIP
    B. Boutonniere deformity—flexion of PIP, extension of DIP
    C. Swan neck deformity—flexion of PIP, extension of DIP
    D. Lanois deformity—medial deviation of digits and dorsal subluxation of MTP joints
    E. Heberdons nodes—soft tissue swelling at dorsal surface of MCP joints

64. **Inflammatory conditions with increased bone scan uptake:**
    A. Cholecystitis   B. Necrotizing enterocolitis
    C. Pneumonia   D. Gout
    E. Abscess

65. **Perifocal bone marrow edema is seen in:**
    A. Stress fracture   B. Osteoid osteoma
    C. Osteochondroma   D. Enchondroma
    E. Histiocytosis

66. **Reiter's disease:**
    A. Metatarsals have fluffy periosteal reaction
    B. HLA B27 patients are affected severely
    C. Related to infective colitis
    D. Affects characteristically, the metacarpophalangeal joints
    E. Symmetrical arthritis

67. **Associations of acromegaly:**
    A. Hypogonadism
    B. Galactorrhoea
    C. Growth hormone suppression
    D. Osteoarthritis
    E. Chondrocalcinosis

68. **Associations of Behçet's syndrome:**
    A. Orogenital ulceration   B. Erythema nodosum
    C. Skin calcification   D. Aneurysms
    E. Knee is the most common joint affected

69. **DISH:**
    A. Causes chondrocalcinosis
    B. In thoracic vertebra, the right side is more affected than the left
    C. Increased incidence in diabetic patients
    D. More common in females
    E. At least 2 vertebrae involved
    F. Disc space reduced

70. **Reactive arthritis:**
    A. Severity parallels that of colitis
    B. Seen in 20% of ulcerative colitis patients
    C. Periarticular osteoporosis is a feature
    D. Seen in 30% of Crohn's disease
    E. Hip joint is the most common site

71. **Radiological features of psoriasis:**
    A. Usually begins before 20 years
    B. Distal phalanges are the most commonly affected
    C. Arthropathy precedes skin lesion
    D. Sacroiliitis is more asymmetrical than Reiter's
    E. Small joints are involved symmetrically

72. **Hemochromatosis arthropathy:**
    A. Chondrocalcinosis is frequent
    B. Osteophytes in interphalangeal joints are typical
    C. Neuropathic changes occur
    D. Subchondral sclerosis is a common finding
    E. Excess copper deposition in the articular cartilage is the
       pathologic finding

73. **Still's disease:**
    A. Delayed skeletal maturation is seen
    B. Hepatosplenomegaly
    C. Large joints affected in pauciarticular form
    D. Early erosive changes in polyarticular form
    E. Equal sex incidence

74. **Wilson's disease:**
    A. Autosomal recessive
    B. Chondrocalcinosis
    C. Squaring of metacarpal heads
    D. Increased sulcal prominence is seen in CT brain
    E. Basal ganglia shows high density regions in cranial CT

75. **Ankylosing spondylitis:**
   A. Unilateral sacroiliitis is an early feature
   B. Symmetrical polyarthritis of large peripheral joints is a typical feature
   C. Periarticular osteopenia is a diagnostic feature
   D. Anderson lesions are painless
   E. Pulmonary fibrosis of upper zones occurs in 15-20%

76. **Seronegative spondyloarthropathy is seen in:**
   A. Ankylosing spondylitis
   B. Rheumatoid arthritis
   C. Behçet's disease
   D. Reiter's disease
   E. Pyogenic arthritis

77. **Ankylosing spondylitis:**
   A. 80% of normal population have HLA B 27 gene
   B. 10% of those with HLA B 27 develop disease
   C. 95% of ankylosing spondylitis patients are HLA B 27 positive
   D. Lower lumbar vertebrae are the earliest affected bones
   E. Degenerative changes are a sequelae of ankylosing spondylitis

78. **Charcots joints:**
   A. Preservation of joint margins
   B. Painful joints are characteristic
   C. Syringomyelia spares lower limb
   D. Knee is the most common site in neurosyphilis
   E. Pencil point deformity of metatarsal heads is seen

79. **Reiter's syndrome:**
   A. Keratoderma blennorrhagica is characteristic
   B. Periosteal new bone formation is characteristic
   C. Urethral discharge is culture positive in 20-30%   ·
   D. Affects lower limbs more frequently than upper limbs
   E. Involves cartilaginous and synovial joints

80. **Radiological changes in neuropathic joint:**
   A. Density decrease   B. Debri
   C. Destruction   D. Distraction
   E. Dislocation

81. **Carpal fusion occurs in:**
   A. Turner's syndrome   B. Still's disease
   C. Psoriasis   D. Arthrogryphosis
   E. Ellis-van Creveld syndrome

82. **Associations of peroneal spastic flat foot:**
    A. Talonavicular fusion
    B. Calcaneonavicular fusion
    C. Tibiofibular synostosis
    D. Appearance of symptoms after 30 years of age
    E. Beaking of head of talus

83. **Narrow posterior end of ribs are seen in:**
    A. Poliomyelitis   B. Pectus excavatum
    C. Tabes dorsalis   D. Rheumatoid arthritis
    E. Neurofibromatosis

84. **Gout:**
    A. Normal X-ray is not seen in presence of severe symptoms
    B. Calcification occurs in joint capsule
    C. Periarticular osteoporosis is characteristic
    D. Fusion of carpal bones is a late phenomenon
    E. Pleural effusion seen after therapy

85. **Sarcoidosis—common features:**
    A. Cortical thickening   B. Lacy pattern
    C. Cortical striations   D. Periosteal reaction
    E. Increased bone density

86. **Sarcoidosis:**
    A. Bone involvement is seen in 15%
    B. Proximal phalanx is the most favoured location
    C. High signal with a serpentine pattern is seen
    D. Non-caesating granulomas
    E. 50% undergoes spontaneous remission

87. **Spondylolisthesis is more common in L4 vertebra because:**
    A. Sagittal orientation of facets at L4-5 level
    B. Bigger transverse process
    C. Restricted mobility
    D. Poor ligamentous support
    E. Firm attachment of lumbosacral joint

88. **Enteropathic arthritis:**
    A. Associated with HLA B 27
    B. Sacroiliitis resolves with colectomy
    C. Peripheral arthritis unchanged by colectomy
    D. Intestinal bypass surgeries cure the disease
    E. Shigella is a cause

ANSWERS

1. **A-T, B-T, C-T, D-T, E-T**
Degenerative subchondral cysts(geode), chondroblastoma and metastasis are other lesions.

2. **A-F, B-F, C-F, D-F, E-T**
Pigmented villonodular synovitis occurs in equal frequency in women and men and occurs in younger age between 20-40 years. The large joints are commonly affected, especially the knee joint. Calcification is uncommon unlike synovial osteochondromatosis and subarticular erosions are seen at the margin of the joints.

3. **A-T, B-F, C-F, D-T, E-T**
There is no periarticular osteoporosis. There is no joint space narrowing in the early stages of PVNS. Soft tissue is dense due to hemosiderin deposit. Hypointence nodules are seen in MRI.

4. **A-F, B-T, C-T, D-F, E-T**
Pathologically pigment may or may not be seen.
Angio is hypervascular and can show AV malformation.
Soft tissue nodules do not calcify. It can extend beyond the capsule of the joint and occasionally can be purely extracapsular. No calcifications.

5. **A-T, B-F, C-T, D-F, E-T**
Other causes of hemarthrosis also cause hemosiderin deposition.

6. **A-T, B-F, C-T, D-F, E-T**
Homocystinuria is radiologically confused with Marfan's syndrome. It has arachnodactyly, kyphoscoliosis, similar to Marfan's syndrome.
Homocystinuria is autosomal recessive. Osteoporosis, Genu valgum, pectus carinatum, deformed teeth, inguinal/umbilical hernia, hypotonia are other findings.
Downward dislocation of lens, articular venous thrombosis are seen.

7. **A-T, B-T, C-T, D-T, E-T**
Juvenile chronic arthritis.

8. **A-F, B-T, C-T, D-T, E-F**
Psoriasis is another common cause.

9. **A-T, B-T, C-T, D-T, E-F**
Psoriasis, scleroderma, multicenteric reticulohistiocytosis are other causes.

10. **A-T, B-F, C-T, D-T, E-T**
Ankylosing spondylitis—is the most common cause.

11. **A-T, B-T, C-F, D-T, E-T**
    Synovial hemangioma—intermediate T1, high T2, low signal septa, vascular channels.

12. **A-F, B-F, C-T, D-T, E-T**
    Juvenile chronic arthritis, pyogenic arthritis, Reiter's, scleroderma are other causes.

13. **A-T, B-F, C-T, D-T, E-T**
    Epidermolysis bullosa—Blister formation in response to mechanical trauma. There are four subtypes. Diagnosis by electron microscopy, immunofluorescence, infections, squamous carcinoma, eye blisters, esophageal structures, malnutrition are complications. Pyloric stenosis, GU obstruction associated.

14. **A-T, B-F, C-F, D-T, E-F**
    Immobilisation, arthroplasty are other causes.

15. **A-F, B-T, C-T, D-T, E-F**
    Isolated fusion involves same row, infections/syndromes—both rows. Idiopathic—females, African, Americans—lunateus triquetrum—most common. Bilateral—60% widening of scapholunate space seen, capitate and hamate is second common. Associated with Holt-Oram, Turner, arthrogryposis, acrocephalosyndactyly, symphalangism.

16. **A-T, B-T, C-T, D-T, E-T**
    Anderson's lesion produces mobility of vertebra at single level and is seen in advanced cases. Carrot stick fracture makes the spine more brittle. Romanus lesion is a erosion seen in the anterioinferior aspect of the vertebral body margin at the site of insertion of annulus fibrosis. Squaring is due to superimposition of anterior periostitis with Romanus lesion.

17. **A-T, B-T, C-F, D-T, E-T**
    Congenital—Aperts, Turner's, Holt-Oram's syndromes, Arthrogryposis congenital multiplex, Ellis-van Creveld syndrome.
    Acquired—RA, JRA, pyogenic, post-traumatic
    Most common is Triquetro—lunate > capitate-hamate > trapezium—trapezoid.

18. **A-F, B-F, C-T, D-T, E-T**
    Upper lobe fibrosis.

19. **A-F, B-T, C-T, D-T, E-T**
    95% have HLA B 27 genotype. 20-50% involvement of peripheral joints, hips, shoulder most common. Sacroiliac joints—bilaterally symmetrical. Initially in lower and middle thirds, more in the iliac

side, subluxation can happen due to fracture of fixed segment. There is association with ankylosing spondylitis, psoriasis, reactive arthritis, inflammatory bowel disease. Fracture spine common in thoracolumbar region.

20. **A-F, B-T, C-T, D-T, E-F**
Restriction of chest expansion is due to ankylosis of costovertebral joints. Peripheral joints, usually hip and knee joints are affected. The visualization of articualr cortex through ankylosed sacroiliac joint is called Ghost sign. Dagger sign is midline ossification in spine due to ossification of interspinous and supraspinous ligaments.

21. **A-T, B-F, C-T, D-T, E-T**
Tachycardia, renal failure due to amyloidosis are other known complications. Initially women bone is deposited in enthesophytes,which is followed by lamellar bone. Synovitis—less severe.

22. **A-T, B-T, C-F, D-F, E-T**
Sclerosis of odontoid is seen after erosions. Hatchet erosions are seen in the supralateral aspect of humerus. Asymmetrical involvement is seen.

23. **A-T, B-T, C-F, D-T, E-T**
Iliac crests, calcaneum, ischial tuberosities, trochanters and spinous processes are commonly affected by enthesopathy. Ankylosis of joint prosthesis occurs in 30-60% of those with ankylosing spondylitis.

24. **A-T, B-T, C-T, D-T, E-F**
CPPD arthropathy, hemophilia, trauma are other causes.

25. **A-T, B-T, C-F, D-T, E-T**
Hypoplastic facets seen in spinal bifida occluta can cause aberrant motion and excessive stress in the neural arch producing pars defects. Napolean's hat sign or Gendarme's cap is seen in L5/S1 spondylolisthesis and is due to superimposition of L5 body and transverse process over S1. Another sign is the Bowline sign of Brailsford.

26. **A-T, B-T, C-T, D-T, E-T**
The Witse classification of spondylolisthesis
I—Dysplastic (Defective development, non-union of 2 centers, genetic)
II—Isthmic(alteration to pars interarticularis articulation). A—lytic or stress fracture of pars, B—elongated pars, C—Acute fracture of pars
III—Degenerative, IV—-Traumatic, V—Pathologic, VI—Postsurgical.

27. **A-T, B-T, C-T, D-T, E-T**
    Spondylolisthesis due to spondylolysis is called true spondylolisthesis and that due to spondylosis is called pseudo. In pseudolisthesis, the steop off is seen below the level of slip. The spinous process of affected level will be as a depression in spondylosis. Hyperlordosis, clicking, hamstring toghness, pelvic waddle, back pain, are other features.

28. **A-T, B-T, C-T, D-T, E-T**
    Other causes are agenesis or hypoplasia of one pedicle or facet, asymmetric facets, metastasis, lymphoma, myeloma, Ewing's, fibrous dysplasia, tuberous sclerosis, arthrodesis, laminectomy, infection. Unilateral spondylolisthesis with compensatory hypertrophy of contralateral pedicle is called Wilkinson syndrome.

29. **A-F, B-T, C-T, D-F, E-T**
    Gaut—30-60 years, Males—9:1. Renal stones, Carpal tunnel syndrome, migratory polyarthritis can be seen. Tophi can be seen in ear helix, olecranon bursa, prepatellar bursa. Tophi calcify very uncommonly. Lower limb is commonly affected, I MTP joint, intertarsal joint, ankles, knees, leukemia, lymphoma, myeloma, other tumors, drugs produce high uric acid and gout.

30. **A-T, B-T, C-T, D-T, E-F**
    Erosions with overhanging edges is the hallmark of disease. Tophi can be seen in joint, periarticular or far away. Soft tissue swelling can be seen anywhere. Joint space loss is very late. There is no loss of bone density. Tophi can be seen inside spinal canal causing cord compression.

31. **A-T, B-T, C-F, D-T, E-F**
    Latent period 5-10 years. Tophi is usually seen in avascular periarticular tissue. Shelf like elevated bony margin is due to bony resorption and deposition. The erosions are usually periarticular, but can be intra-articular or remote from the joint. Effusion, soft tissue swelling earliest.

32. **A-T, B-T, C-T, D-T, E-F**
    Plane joint—intermetatarsal, intercarpal: **Hinge**—humeroulnar, interphalangeal: **Sellar joint**—first capometacarpal, ankle, calcaneocuboid, **Spheroidal joint**—Hip, glenohumeral: **Bicondylar**—Knee, temporomandibular: **Pivot**—Proximal radioulnar, median atlantoaxial: **Hinge**—interphalangeal, Humeroulnar. Knee was considered a hinge joint but has two condylar and an arthrodial joint.

33. **A-F, B-T, C-T, D-T, E-F**

Amniotic bands, also called Streeter's syndrome, is believed to be secondary to premature rupture of amnion with uninjured chorion. This produces raw surfaces that attach and entrap limbs, producing rings of constrictions and amputations of limbs. It is sporadic, more common in first pregnancy, young pregnancies. Associated with club feet, cleft lip and cleft palate. Soft tissue constrictions and amputations of bones are seen in X-rays. It is the most common cause of terminal limb malformation.

34. **A-T, B-T, C-T, D-F, E-F**

Sarcoidosis is the most common cause. Gout, rheumatoid, tuberculosis, Ollier's disease, metastasis, multiple myeloma, hyperparathyroidism, hemangiomas are other causes. Tuberous sclerosis has periosteal reaction, but sarcoidosis does not have periosteal reaction. Ollier's has calcification, bone expansion and endosteal scalloping. Vinyl chloride, epidermolysis bullosa, Acro-osteolysis.

35. **A-T, B-T, C-T, D-T, E-T**

Arthritis can be acute peripheral symmetric polyarthritis affecting small and medium sized joints or chronic polyarthritis affecting large joints and small joints of hands.

36. **A-T, B-T, C-T, D-T, E-F**

Osteoporosis, osteonecrosis, osteomyelitis, fat deposition, soft tissue calcification are other radiological presentations.

37. **A-T, B-F, C-F, D-T, E-F**

Due to infarction of mid-portion of vertebral end plate.

38. **A-F, B-F, C-F, D-T, E-F**

Cupids bow contour refers to the normal concavity on the inferior aspect of lumbar vertebrae. This is best seen in the AP film, and the spinous process forms the bow.

39. **A-F, B-T, C-T, D-F, E-T**

Fish shaped vertebra refers to the typical biconcave appearance of the vertebra. This is caused by diseases producing diffuse weakening of the bone. It is also seen in hyperparathyroidism, renal osteodystrophy and tumours.

40. **A-T, B-F, C-F, D-F, E-T**

Osteoporosis can produce fish shaped vertebra, wedge shaped compression, burst fractures and pancake vertebra due to diffuse flattening. Although both osteoporosis and osteomalacia produce biconcave indentation(fish vertebra), in osteoporosis, the indentation is irregular, superior and inferior end plates are affected unequally. But in osteomalacia, the indentation is smooth, with both superior and inferior end plates affected equally. Compression fractures affect only the anterior column and produce anterior wedging. Burst fractures affect and anterior and middle column (posterior vertebral body). Most of the burst fractures are unstable, with neurological compromise, but some of burst fractures can involve posterior body without neurological symptoms.

41. **A-T, B-F, C-F, D-F, E-F**
Alkaptonuria is asymptomatic in children, but eventually progresses to ochronis and arthropathy in adults. Earliest spinal changes are in the lumbar spine. Discal calcifications occur in the inner fibers of annulus are common in the lumbar level. Cervical spinal involvement is less common. The intervertebral disc spaces are narrowed and vacuum phenomenon is seen.

42. **A-T, B-F, C-F, D-F, E-T**
SLE—Complication—Symmetric, non-erosive, non-deforming polyarthritis (80%), 10% irreversible deformities, carpal irritability, ligamental laxity, insufficiency fractures, infection.
CNS—Vasculopathy, venous thrombosis, abscess, haemorrhage;
Renal—Nephritis, Renal vein thrombosis.
GIT—Esophagial reflux, Ac.cholecystitis, pancreatitis, bowel ischemia
CVS—Vascular, endocarditis, valvulitis, pericarditis, pericardial effusion, myocarditis, pulmonary infection, respiratory muscle dysfunction, pulmonary hypertension, hemorrhage pleural effusion.

43. **A-F, B-F, C-T, D-F, E-F**
Sarcoidosis affects musculoskeletal system in less than 5% of people. It is very uncommon for the musculoskeletal system to be involved without skin or pulmonary involvement. Periosteal reaction is very unusual. Usually sarcoidosis produces osteopenia, coarse striations, punched out cystic lesions or osteosclerosis. Hands are the most common sites to be involved. In the hand the middle and distal phalanges are the most common bones involved, metacarpals and proximal phalanges are occasionally affected.

44. **A-T, B-T, C-T, D-F, E-F**
OA, CPPD, Reiter's, ankylosing spondylitis, neuropathic arthropathy are other causes.

45. **A-T, B-T, C-T, D-T, E-F**
Chondrocalcinosis—Seen in CPPD, Gout, Wilson's disease, acromegaly.

46. **A-T, B-T, C-F, D-F, E-F**
Hemochromatosis—Bone density low, chondrocalcinosis, affects 2nd, 3rd MCP joint, carpometacarpal, intercarpal joints. Joint space narrowing, osteophytes; Dense liver, spleen, Hook-like osteophytes characteristic.

47. **A-T, B-F, C-T, D-T, E-T**
Squamous and adenocarcinoma of the bronchus are more common than the small cell cancer. Skin thickening, hyperhidrosis.

48. **A-T, B-T, C-T, D-T, E-T**
Pulmonary metastasis, pleural fibroma also produce osteoarthropathy. Other rare causes include cystic fibrosis, bronchiectasis, tuberculosis, blastomycosis, pulmonary hemangioma. PCP, Hodgkin's, cirrhosis, ulcerative colitis, Crohn's, amoebic and bacillary dysentery, GI polyps/neoplasm, bowel lymphoma, Whipple, biliary atresia, infected grafts, nasopharyngeal carcinoma, esophageal carcinoma, rib tumours, malignant thymoma, sarcoidosis.

49. **A-T, B-T, C-T, D-T, E-T**
Bone scan shows periarticular uptake due to synovitis Diffuse bilateral uptake is characteristic.
The disease characteristically affects the diaphysis and metaphysis. Tibia and fibula, radius and ulna are the most common ones affected.

50. **A-T, B-F, C-T, D-F, E-T, F-T**
Distal phalanges are affected in 25% of cases. Usually epiphysis spared
Periosteal reaction is smooth initially and become rough later.

51. **A-T, B-F, C-T, D-F, E-T**
Jaccoud's arthropathy is seen in rheumatic heart disease. There is no change in bone density/joint space narrowing/erosion. The salient feature is soft tissue swelling and ulnar deviation and flexion of metacarpophalangeal joints, marked in 4th and 5th finger.

52. **A-F, B-F, C-T, D-F, E-T**
1-5% have splenomegaly.
Felty's syndrome. RA, splenomegaly, neutropenic, pleural effusions —painless/painful men > women, no correlation with arthritis, although almost all with chest findings have it. Manubriosteral joint is synchandrosis, do not affected.
Uveitis, scleritis are also seen.

53. **A-T, B-T, C-F, D-F, E-T**
Soft tissue swelling—capsular distension synovial proliferation. Erosion of ulnar styloid radial styloid, scaphoid are early.

Upper limb and long limb equally affected. Cystic expansion occurs in juvenile arthritis. Fusion is most common in carpals.

54. **A-F, B-T, C-T, D-T, E-F**

55. **A-T, B-T, C-F, D-T, E-F**
Spine cervical spine involved, atlantoaxial junction – most common, IV discs not involved, apophysed joints affected, cervical discs— erosions occurs very late. Fusion occurs.

56. **A-F, B-T, C-T, D-T, E-T**
Protrusio acetabuli is seen in Marfan's syndrome, osteogenesis imperfecta, trauma, rheumatoid, ankylosing spondylitis, Paget's, osteoporosis, osteomalacia and osteoarthritis

57. **A-T, B-T, C-T, D-T, E-T**
Whipple's disease, Crohn's disease, radiotherapy, Rieter's, psoriasis, hyperparathyroidism, paraplegia, gaut, OA are other causes.

58. **A-T, B-T, C-F, D-F, E-T**
Ankylosing spondylitis, gout, CPPD, acromegaly, ochronosis, psoriasis, hyperparathyroidism, rheumatoid and reactive arthritis are bilaterally symmetrical.
Psoriasis, Reiter and Juvenile rheumatoid are bilaterally asymmetrical. Psoriasis is symmetrical/asymmetrical/unilateral.

59. **A-T, B-F, C-T, D-T, E-T**
Bronchoalveolar carcinoma can occur. Distal phalanx, DIP joint affected, CREST (calcinosis, Raynaud's, sclerodactyly, telangiectasia) is seen. Soft tissue atrophy, contractures, calcification, osteopenia, erosion of 1st carpometacarpal joint is characteristic.

60. **A-F, B-F, C-F, D-T, E-T**

61. **A-T, B-T, C-T, D-F, E-F**
Reiter's joint symptoms, arthritis, conjunctivitis (30%). Young males affected, lower limb > upper limb, common in MTP joints and IP joint of great toe, sausage digit, no loss of bone density (except in acute phase) fluffy periosteal reaction, enthesophytes spurs, fusion, sacroiliitis bilaterally asymmetrical, large joints affected in lower limb, uncommon, asymmetrical.

62. **A-F, B-T, C-T, D-F, E-T**
Terry Thomas sign is increases space between scaphoid and lunate and indicates scapholunate dissociation. The cervical spinous process is tapered and called pencil shaped spinous process. In discal involvement there is loss of discal height, but unlike

spodylosis, there are endplate erosions, no sclerosis. The neck length is shorted due to loss of disc height, osteolysis and upward displacement of odontoid process.

63. **A-F, B-T, C-F, D-F, E-F**
Mallet finger—persistent flexion of DIP due to rupture of central slip of extensor digitorum at PIP.
Boutonniére deformity—flexion of PIP, extension of DIP.
Swan neck deformity—extension PIP, flexion DIP.
Lanois deformity—fibular deviation of toes, dorsal subluxation of MTP.
Zig zag deformity—ulnar deviation of fingers, carpal radial rotation.
Haygarth's nodes—soft tissue swelling dorsal to MCP joints.
Heberden's nodes are seen over DIP in osteoarthritis.
Other changs include spindle digit, arthritis mutilans and hitchhikers thumb.

64. **A-F, B-T, C-T, D-T, E-T**

65. **A-T, B-T, C-F, D-F, E-T**

66. **A-T, B-T, C-F, D-F, E-F**
HLA 827 association, more revere, lower limb affected more, asymmetrical.

67. **A-T, B-T, C-F, D-T, E-T**
Acromegaly—Large skull, large sella/sinuses/mandible, hypertrophied extremities, spade like phalanges, hypertrophied articular or cartilage, osteophytes, bone density—normal or low or high, increased helped thickness and sesamoid index; scalloping of vertebral.

68. **A-T, B-T, C-F, D-T, E-T**
Behçet's—Mouth/genital ulcers, iritis, phlebitis, arthritis. Arthritis 60% lower extremities common monoarticular pattern, affecting knee is the most common. Large joints affected, non-deforming, sacroiliitis, aseptic necrosis and entheropathies are seen.

69. **A-T, B-T, C-T, D-F, E-F, F-F**
DISH—Diffuse idiopathic skeletal hyperostosis, men affected more, dorsal spine affected (TT-TII) Left side—less involved due to aortic pulsation (unless right sided aorta); Flowing ossification of at least four contiguous vertebrae, Hyperostosis of ligaments, Disc space—spared; Enthesophytes seen; Sacroiliac joint spared; Recurrent Achilles tendonitis.

70. **A-T, B-T, C-T, D-F, E-F**
20% of UC and 8% of Crohn's are affected. SI joint and spine are commonly affected. Bilaterally symmetrical sacroiliitis,

paravertebral ossification seen soft tissue swelling, osteopenia, synovitis seen.

71. **A-F, B-T, C-F, D-F, E-F**
Psoriasis—Arthropathy in 5% of psoriasis; 70% pauciarticular, 15% like RA, 5% DIP, spondylitis, arthritis mutilans, skin lesions usually seen. Sacroiliitis-bilaterally symmetrical in 50%; 35-55 years; small joints asymmetrical.

72. **A-T, B-F, C-T, D-F, E-F**
60% have chondrocalcinosis. Osteophytes are characteristically seen in the metatarsophalangeal joints of middle and ring fingers. Neuropathic changes are seen in later stages due to diabetes. Subchondral sclerosis is rare. Excess iron deposition is the characteristic finding.

73. **A-F, B-T, C-T, D-F, E-F**
Accelerated skeletal maturation is seen due to hyperemia. Felty's disease is associated with arthritis, hepatosplenomegaly and leucopenia. Ankles, knees and wrists are common joints involved in pauciarticular form. Erosive changes are uncommon and late. Males are affected five times as common as females.

74. **A-T, B-T, C-F, D-T, E-F**
Squaring of metacarpal heads is a feature of hemochromatosis. Atrophic changes are common. Low density lesions are seen in basal ganglia.

75. **A-F, B-F, C-F, D-F, E-F**
Usually bilateral sacroiliitis is seen. Asymmetrical involvement of large joints.
Osteopenia is rare. Anderson' lesions are stress fractures and are painful.
Upper lobe fibrosis is seen in 1%.

76. **A-T, B-F, C-F, D-T, E-F**
Ankylosing spondylitis, Psoriasis, Reiter's disease, Reactive arthritis and undifferentiated spondyloarthropathy are sero-negative spondyloarthropathy.

77. **A-T, B-F, C-T, D-F, E-T**
80% of normal population have HLA B 27. Only 2% of those with HLA B 27 develop the disease. 90-95% of those with ankylosing spondylitis have HLA B 27 gene. Sacroiliac joints are the earliest affected region in AS. Degenerative changes are a long-term sequelae due to restricted mobility.

78. **A-F, B-F, C-T, D-T, E-T**
Neuropathic joints are due to loss of joint sensation are due to local hyperemia and bone destruction.

DM—Foot (MTP, TM, Intertarial), Tabes—knee, hip, ankle, spine, leprosy (hand feet), syringomyelia (shoulder, upper limb), Alcohol (MTP, IP joints), Congenital insensity to pain, fragmentation of articular margins/subluxations dislocations debris, sclerosis.

79. **A-T, B-T, C-F, D-T, E-T**
Urethral cultures are negative; entheropathy seen.

80. **A-F, B-T, C-T, D-F, E-T**
Density increase, debri, destruction, dislocation and disorganisation are the five Ds associated with Charcots joint.

81. **A-F, B-T, C-F, D-T, E-T**

82. **A-T, B-T, C-F, D-F, E-F**
Peroneal spastic flat foot has flat foot and short peroneal muscles, producing pain on attempted inversion. Can be acquired, due to trauma, JRA, infection.

83. **A-T, B-F, C-F, D-T, E-T**

84. **A-F, B-T, C-F, D-F, E-F**
X-ray can be normal in acute stages; normal bone density, no carpal fusion.

85. **A-F, B-T, C-T, D-F, E-F**
The bone density is decreased and the cortex is thinned. Striations may be seen in cortex.
Cystic lesions in a lacy pattern are seen. Periosteal reaction is very uncommon.
Increased bone density is occasionally seen but it is not a common feature.

86. **A-F, B-T, C-T, D-T, E-T**
Bone is involved in 5% of sarcoidosis. Middle and distal phalanx are commonly affected. High signal in T2, low signal in T1, with serpentine and target patern are characteristic.

87. **A-T, B-F, C-F, D-T, E-T**
The facets are oriented in a sagittal plane in L4/5. This places a lot of stress on the joint, added to the fact that lumbosacral joint is fixed . The transverse process of L4 is small and is more mobile.

88. **A-T, B-F, C-F, D-F, E-T**
Sixty percent association with HLAB27. Shigella, salmonella, campylobacter, yersinia, clostridium difficile, strongyloides, Taenia saginata, gardia, ascaris, cryptosporidism, UC, Crohn's Whipple's, celiac disease, collagenous colitis, intestinal bypass surgery are other causes. Peripheral arthritis resolves with colectomy, spondylitis and sacroiliitis do not resolve.

3 Infection

1. **Osteomyelitis and the most common organisms:**
   A. Newborns—*Pseudomonas*
   B. Children—*E. coli*
   C. Adults—*Staphylococcus aureus*
   D. Drug adicts—*Klebsiella*
   E. Sickle cell—*Streptococcus*

2. **Osteomyelitis:**
   A. Genitourinary tract infection is the most common cause of osteomyelitis
   B. Common in lower limb than upper limb
   C. Lumbar vertebrae are commonly affected than thoracic vertebrae
   D. Direct implantation from trauma is the most common cause
   E. Fever and raised white cells are seen in two-thirds

3. **Complications of osteomyelitis:**
   A. Amyloidosis
   B. Squamous cell carcinoma
   C. Fistula
   D. Limb length discrepancy
   E. Osteopathia striata

4. **Nuclear medicine in osteomyelitis:**
   A. Gallium scan is positive only after the MDP scan is positive
   B. Gallium is very useful in chronic osteomyelitis
   C. Cold spot excludes osteomyelitis
   D. False negative rate higher in children
   E. Cellulitis cannot be differentiated from osteomyelitis

5. **Lesions producing the same appearance as osteomyelitis in bone scan:**
   A. Paget's disease   B. Septic arthritis
   C. Diabetic neuropathy   D. Tumours
   E. Post-traumatic

6. **White cell scans in osteomyelitis:**
   A. Initial cold area becomes hot in vertebra
   B. In 111 labelled leukocytes is the best for acute infection
   C. Tc 99m labelled leukocytes preferred for extremities
   D. WBC scan is better than gallium scans
   E. Uptake is increased within 24 hours

7. **Terms used in osteomyelitis:**
   A. Cloaca—layer of living bone formed about the dead bone
   B. Involucrum—opening in the cloaca through which the granulation tissue comes out
   C. Garré's osteomyelitis—non purulent
   D. Osteitis—only the cortex is affected
   E. Sequestrum—Denser than normal bone

8. **The following are causes of paraplegia in tuberculosis:**
   A. Endarteritis
   B. Intramedullary granuloma
   C. Arachnoiditis
   D. Vascular malformation due to pressure of bone
   E. Pathological fracture

9. **Brodie's abscess:**
   A. Lower limb is the most common site
   B. Extension never occurs into the epiphysis
   C. Eccentric in 10% of cases
   D. Sclerotic margin is common
   E. Majority of patients are older than 40

10. **Brodie's abscess:**
    A. Serpiginous channel extending towards growth plate is pathognomonic
    B. Periosteal reaction excludes Brodie's abscess
    C. MRI shows an inner high signal and outer high signal in T2W images
    D. Tuberculosis is the most common organisms causing this
    E. If left untreated results in sclerosing osteomyelitis of Garré

11. **Tuberculosis arthritis:**
    A. Joint is usually affected secondary to bone involvement
    B. 30% is seen in extrapulmonary tuberculosis
    C. High glucose in joint fluid
    D. Cartilage destruction is faster than in pyogenic
    E. No osteoporosis

12. **Septic arthritis:**
    A. Gonorrhoea is a causative organism
    B. *Staphylococcus* is the most common organism
    C. *Salmonella* is the most common organism in children before four years
    D. Causes osteoarthritis
    E. Avacular necrosis is a sequelae

13. **Septic arthritis:**
    A. Joint space narrowing is very rapid
    B. Joint effusion is the first sign in X-ray
    C. Metaphyseal bone is destroyed
    D. No sclerosis in underlying bone
    E. Erosions are marginal

14. **Complications of septic arthritis:**
    A. Synovial cyst
    B. Widening of joint space
    C. Avascular necrosis
    D. Transient regional osteoporosis
    E. Resorption of sesamoid bones

15. **Tuberculosis:**
    A. If skin test is not positive, diagnosis is excluded
    B. Active pulmonary disease is seen in 50%
    C. Most common location is the hip
    D. Reactivation is most common in the hip
    E. Can be formed from an extraosseous focus

16. **The following are features of tuberculous than pyogenic spondylitis:**
    A. Multiple level involvement
    B. Rapid destruction
    C. Sclerosis
    D. Involvement of posterior elements
    E. Calcified abscess cavity

17. **Tuberculous arthritis:**
    A. Bony ankylosis is the end result
    B. Synovial biopsy is positive in 50% of cases
    C. Marginal erosions are seen
    D. Phemisters triad is characteristic
    E. Draining sinus is not seens in pyogenic osteomyelitis

18. **Radiology of acute osteomyelitis:**
    A. X-rays normal for three weeks in axial skeleton
    B. Soft tissue swelling is the earliest finding
    C. Bone changes are seen only when 50% of bone is involved
    D. X-ray changes of bone destruction are behind the pathological changes by two weeks
    E. Periosteal reaction develops after 20 days

19. **Tuberculous arthritis:**
    A. Joint effusion is seen in majority of hip joint arthritis
    B. Marginal erosions are more common in the non-weight bearing aspect of the joints
    C. Cortical bone destruction is earlier in hip joints
    D. Joint space narrowing is seen within days of onset
    E. Kissing sequestrum are seen

20. **Tuberculous osteomyelits:**
    A. Rare in adults
    B. Epiphysis is not commonly involved
    C. Do not extend across the physis
    D. Epiphyseal focus spreads to the joint
    E. Sclerosis is seen around the lytic lesion

21. **TB spine:**
    A. 25-50% of skeletal tuberculosis
    B. Dorsolumbar vertebra are the commonly affected
    C. Posterior elements are commonly involved
    D. Starts in the anterioinferior aspect of the vertebra
    E. Multiple levels are commonly involved

22. **TB spine:**
    A. Subligamentous spread produces anterior scalloping
    B. The earliest change is presence of paravertebral soft tissue
    C. Vertebral disc space earlier than in pyogenic spondylitis
    D. Calcified paravertebral mass is pathognomonic
    E. Hematogenous spread is via Batson's plexus

23. **The following are radiological features of TB spine:**
    A. Ivory vertebra   B. Vertebra within vertebra
    C. Picture frame vertebra D. Vertebra plana
    E. Romanu's lesion

24. **Complications of tuberculous spine:**
    A. Osteonecrosis
    B. Spinal cord compression
    C. Kyphosis
    D. Arachnoiditis
    E. Ankylosis

25. **TB spine:**
    A. Soft tissue is seen in 50% of tuberculous spondylitis
    B. Soft tissue is not seen without bone destruction
    C. Retropharyngeal abscess is a complication of cervical spinal tuberculosis
    D. Spread by the subligamentous route is specific to tuberculosis
    E. In paraplegic patients, the vertebrae are smaller than normal,

26. **Transient synovitis of hip:**
    A. Most common non-traumatic cause of limp in children
    B. History of recent viral disease in majority
    C. X-ray shows erosion on the head of the femur
    D. Lateral displacement of the gluteal fat pad is the most sensitive method for diagnosis
    E. Osteoporosis is not a feature

27. **Tuberculous osteomyelitis:**
    A. Periosteal reaction is of onion skin type
    B. Epiphyseal overgrowth is a complication
    C. Cystic tuberculosis is common in the shoulder
    D. Cystic tuberculosis has a rim of sclerosis in adults
    E. No periosteal reaction is seen around spina ventosa

28. **Leprosy:**
    A. Periosteitis is seen in 5% of leprosy patients
    B. Metaphysis is the site preferentially involved
    C. Phalanges are commonly involved than metatarsals
    D. Arthritis commonly involves the wrist more commonly than ankle
    E. They are prone for pyogenic osteomyelitis

29. **Leprosy:**
    A. Sacroiliitis is a recognized feature
    B. Index finger is the most common bone involved
    C. Separation of forefoot and hindfoot
    D. Licked candy stick appearance is due to absorption of bones
    E. Distal phalanges are preferentially resorbed in foot

30. **Tuberculosis of spine:**
    A. Most common site of skeletal TB
    B. Rarely involves the neural arch
    C. Affects body of vertebra in 50-60% of cases
    D. Has a very poor prognosis
    E. Typically erodes the spinous end plates

31. **Bone scan:**
    A. Osteomyelitis may be cold
    B. Myocardial infarction is hot
    C. Lytic phase of Paget's disease is cold
    D. 10% of metastases appear cold
    E. Fibrous dysplasia is cold

32. **Osteitis pubis:**
    A. Bilaterally symmetrical
    B. X-rays help differentiating from osteomyelitis
    C. Pelvic surgery is the most common cause in males
    D. Common in athletes
    E. Degree of uptake in bone scan correlates with the severity of disease

33. **Differential diagnosis for lytic lesions in the pubic symphysis:**
    A. Psoriasis
    B. Hyperparathyroidism
    C. Ankylosing spondylitis
    D. Rheumatoid
    E. Reiter's

34. **Brucellosis:**
    A. There is no risk of infection by direct contact
    B. Multiple vertebral involvement is uncommon
    C. Sclerosis is more than that in tuberculosis
    D. Abscess formation is as common as in tuberculosis
    E. Exuberant osteophyte formation is a feature.

ANSWERS

1. **A-F, B-F, C-T, D-F, E-F**
   Newborns—Staph, *E. coli*, Group B Streptococcus, Children—Staph
   Adults, Staph: Drug addicts—Pseudomonas, Sickle—Salmonella.

2. **A-T, B-T, C-T, D-F, E-T**
   Infection is spread by hematogenous or direct implantation or from
   adjacent structures. Hematogenous is common.
   The focus can come either from genitourinary infection or lung
   infection or skin infection.

3. **A-T, B-T, C-T, D-T, E-F**
   Limb length discrepancy is due to epiphyseal hyperemia in
   children. Fracture, arthritis, extension into surrounding structures
   are other complications. Carcinoma is seen in 0.5% of cases and
   are seen deep inside the wound tract.

4. **A-F, B-T, C-F, D-T, E-F**
   Gallium scan is positive a day earlier than Tc MDP scan. Cold spot
   can be seen in osteomyelitis due to vascular occlusion. False
   negative rate in children is higher due to normal uptake in
   epiphysis, where lesions can be missed. Cellulitis shows increased
   uptake in the angiography and blood pool phase, but the static
   images will not show increased uptake.

5. **A-T, B-T, C-T, D-T, E-T**
   Osteomyelitis can produce hot or cold spot and the appearances
   are nonspecific.
   Bone scan has a 92% sensitivity but 87% specificity.

6. **A-F, B-T, C-T, D-T, E-T**
   WBC scans are better than gallium scans because of lesser dose,
   faster imaging and better resolution. Uptake is seen in 24-72 hours.

7. **A-F, B-F, C-T, D-T, E-T**
   Sequestrum—segment of necrotic bone separated form living bone
   by granulation tissue.
   Involucrum—layer of living bone formed about the sequestrum.
   Cloaca—opening in involucrum, through which granulation tissue
   comes out.

8. **A-T, B-T, C-T, D-F, E-F**
   Bone fragments, granulation tissue and abscess are other causes
   of paraplegia in tuberculosis.

9. **A-T, B-F, C-T, D-T, E-F**
   Tibia and femur are the most common locations. Epiphyseal extension occurs, especially in children. A rind of sclerosis is a characteristic feature. It is more common in children.

10. **A-T, B-F, C-T, D-F, E-F**
    The characteristic appearance is a lucent lesion surrounded by a rind of sclerosis. There may be associated periosteal reaction and soft tissue swelling. MRI shows an inner high signal due to granulation tissue and outer low signal of sclerosis in T2W images. Staphylococcus is the most common organism. Sclerosing osteomyelitis of Garré is a separate entity.

11. **A-T, B-T, C-F, D-F, E-F**
    Usually joint involvement is secondary to adjacent bone involvement. Joint fluid shows low glucose, high white cells and low mucin formation. Cartilage destruction is faster in pyogenic.Osteoporosis is a salient feature of tuberculous arthritis.

12. **A-T, B-T, C-F, D-T, E-T**
    Staphylococcus aureus is the most common organism in children over four years and adults.
    In children less than four years, Streptococcus pyogenes is the most common organism.

13. **A-T, B-F, C-T, D-F, E-F**
    In pyogenic arthritis, the joint space narrowing is more rapid, there is sclerosis in the underlying bone and erosions are not marginal. Metaphyseal bone is destroyed due to spread of infection or if infection spread from here. Soft tissue swelling develops before joint effusion and manifested by displacement of fat planes.

14. **A-T, B-T, C-T, D-F, E-T**
    Synovial cyst can rupture and form sinus tract. Other complcations include soft tissue and tendon injury, boney ankylosis, osteomyelitis, degeneration, epiphyseal displacement, epiphyseal enlargement, abscesses .

15. **A-F, B-T, C-F, D-T, E-T**
    Most common location is the spine. The disease is produced by hematagenous dissemination of pulmonary or extrapulmonary focus. Skin test positive—85-95%. Negative in HIV.

16. **A-F, B-F, C-F, D-T, E-T**
    Multiple level involvement can be seen in both. Rapid destruction, sclerosis, involvement of posterior elements, multiple abscess cavities without calcification are all features of pyogenic

spondylitis. Tuberculosis usually produces lysis and osteopenia, but can produce sclerosis in blacks. Paraspinal mass is large and out of proportion to the discovertebral lesion. It is small and not calcifed in pyogenic infections. Whereas pyogenic is diffuse, tuberculosis is segmental and of insidious onset.

17. **A-F, B-F, C-T, B-T, E-F**
Tuberculous arthritis ends in fibrous ankylosis, unlike pyogenic which ends in bony ankylosis. Synovial biopsy is positive in 90%. Phemisters triad is joint space narrowing, marginal erosions and osteoporosis. Soft tissue swelling and draining sinus are seen in both.

18. **A-T, B-T, C-T, D-T, E-T**
X-ray changes are seen after 10 days in appendicular skeleton and after 21 days in axial skeleton. Soft tissue swellling 3-10 days. Periosteal reaction—20 days. Sequestrum-30 days. Sequestrum is necrotic bone. Cloaca is the space where the necrotic bone is placed.

19. **A-F, B-T, C-T, D-F, E-T**
Joint effusion is a common feature, but is not frequently ₃een in hip joint. Cortical bone destruction is earlier in joints with more opposed surfaces, such as hip and knee.
Joint space narrowing takes a long time. Kissing sequestrum is due to destruction on both sides of the joint.

20. **A-T, B-F, C-F, D-T, E-F**
Tuberculosis is common in children. Epiphysis and metaphysis are commonly involved.They cross the physis, unlike pyogenic osteomyelitis. The lytic lesion does not have a rim of sclerosis.

21. **A-T, B-T, C-F, D-T, E-T**
L1 is the common vertebra involved. The body is commonly involved than the posterior elements. Pulmonary lesions are not seen in the majority of patients.

22. **A-T, B-F, C-F, D-T, E-T**
Tuberculous focus may reach the spine either via bloodstream through the Batson's plexus or lymphatics or from contiguous structures. The earliest change is erosion of end plate, which starts at the anterioinferior portion of the subchondral bone (called as the gouge defect). Vertebral disc space is preserved unlike pyogenic spondylitis, where it is destroyed earlier. Calcified paravertebral soft tissue as in psoas, is very characteristic.

23. **A-T, B-T, C-F, D-T, E-F**
Ivory vertebra is also seen in Paget's, lymphoma and metastasis and is seen due to revascularisation and reossification. Vertebra

within vertebra is due to growth recovery lines. Picture frame vertebra is seen in Paget's disease. Vertebra plana is due to collapse of vertebra and seen in children. The most common lesion is eosinophilic granuloma.

Romanu's lesion is seen in ankylosing spondylitis

24. **A-T, B-T, C-T, D-T, E-T**
Paraplegia is a common complication either due to abscess or granulation tissue or arachnoiditis.

25. **A-F, B-F, C-T, D-T, E-F**
Soft tissue is seen only in 5% of those with tuberculosis and is common in the dorsolumbar region. Soft tissue is often out of proportion to the bony and discal lesions and can be seen without any discal or bony change. It is psoas abscess in the abdomen, paravertebral abscess in the thorax and retropharyngeal abscess in the cervical region. The subligamentous spread produces a defect in the anterior concave border of the vertebra called the gouge defect. In paraplegic patient, the vertebra is taller than it is borad and this is due to increased biomechanical stress placed on the vertebral body immediately caudal to gibbus.

26. **A-T, B-T, C-F, D-F, E-F**
X-ray is normal. Osteoporosis can be seen. The main finding is effusion in the joint. This can be demonstrated by displacement of fat pads around the hip joint, of which the gluteal pad is the least sensitive. Diagnosis from other diseases is one of exclusion and it is managed by stopping weight bearing.

27. **A-F, B-T, C-T, D-T, E-F**
Accelerated growth can be seen due to epiphyseal hyperemia. Cystic tuberculosis is common in skull, shoulder and pelvis. It has a rim of sclerosis in adults but not in children. It is seen along the long axis of the bone, round and small, with well-defined sclerotic margins. In children, symmetrical metaphyseal involvement is seen.

Spina ventosa is tuberculosis of digits. This is characterised by expansile lesion, with periosteal reaction.

28. **A-T, B-T, C-T, D-F, E-T**
Lupus periostitis is due to presence of bacilli from overlying dermal or mucosal infection. Soft tissue swelling, osteoporosis, endosteal thining, osseous destruction, pathological fracture, epiphyseal collapse and deformity are common manifestations. Arthritis commonly involves the ankle > knee > wrist > finger.

29. **A-T, B-T, C-T, D-T, E-F**

    Neuropathic arthropathy is one of the most common manifestations of leprosy and is commonly seen in the foot. There is resorption of cancellous bone and concentric atrophy of the bone producing tapered ends also called the licked candy stick appearance. There is preferential resorption of proximal phalanges and metatarsals in feet and distal phalanges in hand . There is tarsal disintegration resulting in separation of forefoot and hindfoot, with osteolysis, osteosclerosis, fragmentation and resorption. Tibia is driven downwards and becomes the weight bearing bone.

30. **A-T, B-T, C-F, D-T, E-T**

    50% of skeletal lesions are seen in the spine. Neural arch is not involved commonly
    Body is involved in 80% has a mortality of 25%.

31. **A-T, B-T, C-F, D-T, E-T**

    Paget's is hot in lytic phase.

32. **A-T, B-F, C-T, D-T, E-F**

    Osteitis pubis is inflammation of pubic symphysis/surrounding muscle insertions.
    In males, pelvic surgery for prostate and bladder and sports are most common causes. In females, vaginal delivery or pelvic surgery are common causes. It is usually bilateral.
    X-ray shows subchondral irregularity. Increased uptake is seen in bone scan, but it does not correlate with the disease severity.

33. **A-T, B-T, C-T, D-F, E-F**

    Trauma, osteitis, osteomyelitis are other common causes.

34. **A-F, B-F, C-F, D-F, E-T**

    Brucellosis is caused by infection with Brucella melitensis/suis/abortis. Usually infection is obtained by consumption of contaminated milk. But direct contact is a mode of infection, especially in farm workers and abattoir workers. Multiple vertebral involvement is common. Tuberculosis is the most common differential diagnosis. Sclerosis is more common than in tuberculosis but abscess formation is less. Osteophyte formation and fusion are seen in chronic stages.

4 Systemic and Metabolic Disease

1. **Osteoporosis:**
   A. Fractures of the spine are the most serious
   B. 20% of those with hip fractures die within one year
   C. X-ray is sensitive in detection of bone density
   D. BMD must be decreased by 20% before it is radiographically detectable
   E. The number of osteoporotic fractures is expected to decrease in the future due to early diagnosis and new drugs

2. **Techniques very useful in detection of bone mass density:**
   A. Single X-ray absorptiometry
   B. Dual X-ray absorptiometry
   C. Quantitative ultrasound
   D. Quantitative computed tomography
   E. Quantitative MRI

3. **Transient regional osteoporosis of hip:**
   A. More common in the right side
   B. Seen in third trimester of pregnancy
   C. Males are never affected
   D. Swelling of joint is seen clinically
   E. Very slow progression

4. **Transient osteoporosis of hip:**
   A. Joint space narrowing is seen in the late stages
   B. Collapse of subchondral bone
   C. Cold spot in bone scan
   D. MRI the most sensitive
   E. Pathological fracture is not a feature

5. **Regional migratory osteoporosis:**
   A. Joint space narrowed if the disease is progressive
   B. Lasts for 6-9 months in a joint
   C. High signal in T2W MRI
   D. Bone erosion
   E. Middle aged males commonly affected

6. **Foreign body in soft tissue:**
   A. Wood is not echogenic in ultrasound
   B. CT is superior than ultrasound for superficial non-radiopaque foreign bodies
   C. A hypoechoic rim around the foreign body suggests an alternate diagnosis
   D. Posterior shadowing depends on the composition of the foreign body
   E. Glass usually produces clean posterior acoustic shadowing

7. **Tarsal tunnel components:**
   A. Flexor digitorum longus tendon
   B. Tibialis anterior tendon
   C. Flexor hallucis longus tendon
   D. Extensor hallucis longus tendon
   E. Posterior tibal nerve

8. **Diabetic foot:**
   A. Neuropathic changes commonly involve the metatarsophalangeal joints
   B. Presence of pain excludes neuropathic joints
   C. Neuropathic joints produce low signal in T1 and high signal in T2, but do not enhance like osteomyelitis
   D. Septic arthritis is most common in the tarsometatarsal joints
   E. Ulcers are most common under the second and third metatarsal heads

9. **The following findings favour osteomyelitis rather than neuropathic joint:**
   A. Sinus tract
   B. Interruption of cortex
   C. Fragmented bone
   D. Increased density
   E. Joint space reduction

10. **Gout:**
    A. Always located in a periarticular location
    B. Tophi enhance on gadolinium MRI
    C. Tophi have low signal in T1 and T2
    D. Causes bursitis
    E. Elicits granulomatous reaction in chronic cases

11. **Hypercalcemia associated with:**
    A. Paget's disease   B. Fibrous dysplasia
    C. Multiple myeloma   D. CA bronchus
    E. Sarcoidosis

12. **Lesions causing hypercalcemia:**
    A. Pancreatitis
    B. Myeloma
    C. Sarcoidosis
    D. Ochronosis
    E. Cysticercosis

13. **Paget's disease:**
    A. Spine and skull are the commonly affected bones
    B. Bone scans are required to differentiate from metastatic disease
    C. Fibrosarcoma is the important complication
    D. Vascular calcification is a consequence of increased bone turnover
    E. Renal stones are associated

14. **Avascular necrosis of femoral head occurs in:**
    A. Thalassemia
    B. Chronic alcoholism
    C. Cushing's syndrome
    D. Gaucher's disease
    E. Congenital dislocation of hip

15. **The following have high serum calcium and high alkaline phosphatase:**
    A. Hyperthyroidism
    B. Hypoparathyroidism
    C. Metastasis
    D. Multiple myeloma
    E. Paget's disease

16. **Hypophosphatasia features:**
    A. Rachitic changes
    B. Renal calculi
    C. Phosphoethanolamine in urine
    D. Normal skull sutures
    E. Basal ganglia calcification

17. **Paget's disease:**
    A. High output cardiac failure is a recognized complication
    B. Sarcoma occurs in 20% of cases
    C. Bone pain is relieved by calcitonin
    D. Serum alkaline phosphatase is depressed
    E. Paraplegia is a recognized complication

18. **Transient osteoporosis of hip:**
    A. The intertrochanteric region of femur shows high signal in MRI commonly
    B. Recurs in another joint in 2 years
    C. Recovery takes 3-6 weeks
    D. Can be confused with avascular necrosis
    E. Rheumatoid arthritis is a differential diagnosis

19. **Regional migratory osteoporosis:**
    A. Pain on weight bearing
    B. Common in the upper limb, unliked transient osteoporosis of hip
    C. Osteopororis seen in 4 months after onset
    D. Spares the trabecular bone
    E. Periosteal reaction is seen

20. **Paget's disease:**
    A. Affects any bone
    B. Equally seen in men and women
    C. Acid phosphatase levels in blood is raised
    D. Sarcomatous changes is very common
    E. Bi concave vertebra is the most common vertebral finding

21. **Paget's disease:**
    A. Lytic phase is a contraindication to calcitonin therapy
    B. Hot spot in bone scan will decrease in activity after calcitonin
    C. Cervical cord compression is a contraindication to calcitonin therapy
    D. Spinal cord compression is most common at lumbar level
    E. Deafness is due to Pagetoid involvement of ossicles

22. **Paget's disease:**
    A. Osteoporosis circumscripta starts in the parietal bones
    B. Femoral fractures are subtrochanteric
    C. Alkaline phosphase falls if sarcoma develop
    D. Serum calcium is elevated in uncomplicated cases
    E. Incremental fractures are seen in the medial side of the neck of femur

23. **Paget's disease is associated with:**
    A. Enlarged pituitary fossa
    B. Cardiac enlargment
    C. Bone sarcoma
    D. Absence of frontal sinuses
    E. Aneurysm of middle meningeal artery

24. **The association of skin and bone lesion and diabetes insipidus is seen in:**
    A. Histiocytosis
    B. Amyloidosis
    C. Neurofibromatosis
    D. Chronic renal failure
    E. Sarcoidosis

25. **Avascular necrosis occurs in:**
    A. Thalassemia
    B. Alcoholism
    C. Acute pancreatitis
    D. Hypercholesterolemia
    E. Polycythemia rubra vera

26. **Avascular necrosis is a feature of:**
    A. Scaphoid fracture
    B. Humeral neck fracture
    C. Olecranon fractrure
    D. Femoral neck fracture
    E. Talar fracture

27. **Avascular necrosis:**
    A. Avascular necrosis of scaphoid is common with proximal than waist fractures
    B. Avascular necrosis of lunate is more common in manual workers
    C. Severe osteoarthritis causes rotatory subluxation of the scaphoid
    D. Fractured scaphoid is not hot on bone scan until 1 week post injury
    E. After renal transplantation, usually occurs within two years

28. **Osteochondritis dissecans:**
    A. Plain film always identifies the loose body
    B. Can occur in the ankle
    C. Involvement of both knees is rare
    D. Commonly causes loose body in the knee of a young adult
    E. With time separate bony fragments will disappear

29. **Avascular necrosis of hip:**
    A. 70% of contralateral hip is affected
    B. 25% of traumatic avascular necrosis is due to dislocation
    C. Increased density in bone is due to new bone deposition
    D. Joint space is narrowed
    E. Subchondral crescent is seen in the anteriosuperior portion of femoral head

30. **MRI in avascular necrosis:**
    A. In late stages, there is enhancement around the subcondral fracture cleft
    B. Contrast enhancement is seen at interface of lesion and surrounding marrow
    C. Pseudohomogenous edema produces low signal in T1
    D. Fracture cleft shows low signal in both T1 and T2
    E. Coronal images are the best

31. **Differential diagnosis for femoral head irregularity and collapse:**
    A. Sickle cell disease
    B. Meyer's dysplasia
    C. Gaucher's
    D. Hemophilia
    E. Spondyloepiphyseal dysplasia

32. **Recognised complications of Perthes' disease:**
    A. Recurrence
    B. Osteochondritis dissecans
    C. Acute chondrolysis
    D. Large femoral head
    E. Osteoporosis

33. **The following factors are bad risk factors in prognosis of Perthes' disease:**
    A. Males
    B. Early age of onset
    C. Horizontal orientation of growth plate
    D. Lateral epiphysis situated outside the acetabular rim
    E. Early closure of growth plate

34. **Avascular necrosis:**
    A. In stage A, signal is similar to that of fat
    B. In stage C, low signal is seen in both T1
    C. Sclerosis is the earliest finding in stage I of disease
    D. Joint space narrowing in stage III
    E. Subchondral fracture occurs in stage III

35. **Kienböck's disease:**
    A. More common in the left hand
    B. 75% have negative ulnar variance
    C. 20-40 years
    D. Managed conservatively
    E. Venous congestion is a probable cause

36. **Kienböck's disease:**
    A. MRI is normal in stage I
    B. Flattening of radial border in stage II
    C. Joint instability in stage II
    D. Degenerative changes in stage V
    E. Complete collapse in stage III

37. **Complications of Kienböck's disease:**
    A. Perilunate dislocation
    B. Scapholunate separation
    C. Ulnar devation of triquetrum
    D. Degeneration of radiocarpal compartment
    E. Degeneration of midcarpal joint

38. Causes of spontaneous osteonecrosis of knee:
   A. Meniscal tear
   B. Rheumatoid
   C. Gout
   D. Chondromalacia
   E. Osteoarthritis

39. Spontaneous osteonecrosis of knee:
   A. Common in the second decade
   B. Bone scan is positive within five weeks
   C. Flattened lateral femoral condyle
   D. Periosteal reaction along medial side of femoral head
   E. Osteochondral fragment is seen in 9 months

40. Osteomalacia presenting in later life may be due to:
   A. Paget's disease
   B. Pancreatic disease
   C. Idiopathic steatorrhoea
   D. Tuberous sclerosis
   E. Hunter-Hurler syndrome

41. Progressive myositis ossificans:
   A. Associated with Raynaud's phenomenon
   B. Associated with occular malignant neoplasm
   C. Associated with short first metacarpal
   D. Onset in middle age
   E. Associated with nephrocalcinosis

42. Avascular necrosis is seen in:
   A. Gaucher's disease
   B. Niemann-Pick disease
   C. Diver's
   D. Pregnancy
   E. Frostbite

43. Features of hypothyroidism:
   A. Wormian bones
   B. Widening of intervertebral space
   C. Bullet shaped vertebra
   D. Metaphyseal bands
   E. Pseudo-obstruction

44. Associations of thyroid acropachy:
   A. Grave's disease   B. Hashimoto's disease
   C. Papillary carcinoma   D. Exophthalmos
   E. Pretibial myxedema

45. **Features of thyroid acropachy:**
    A. Fusiform proximal phalanges
    B. Lamellar periosteal new bone formation along the metacarpals
    C. Affects long bones
    D. Marked thickening of overlying skin
    E. Short fifth metacarpal

46. **Thyroid acropachy:**
    A. Periosteal reaction is characteristically seen in the metaphyseal region
    B. Periosteal reaction is bilaterally symmetrical
    C. Spiculated periosteal reaction is seen
    D. Clubbing is associated
    E. Erosion of the corner of metaphysis are a recognised feature

47. **Features of hypopituitarism:**
    A. Large sella
    B. Unfused epiphysis
    C. Wormian bones
    D. Hypoplastic sinuses
    E. Osteopenia

48. **Radiological features of hyperthyroidism:**
    A. Osteopenia
    B. Accelerated growth of osssification centers
    C. Cardiomegaly
    D. Thymic atrophy
    E. Cortical striation

49. **Radiological features of myxedema:**
    A. Pericardial effusion   B. Gastric dilatation
    C. Pseudo-obstruction   D. Pneumonia
    E. Wormian bones

50. **Radiological features of Cushing's syndrome:**
    A. Vertebral wedging
    B. Rib fractures
    C. Decreased callus formation
    D. Wormian bones
    E. Kyphosis

51. **Fluoride levels and disease:**
    A. Normal is less than 1 ppm
    B. 4 ppm—skeletal fluorosis
    C. 6 ppm—dental mottling
    D. 10 ppm—growth disturbance
    E. 15 mm—osteosclerosis

52. Fluorosis:
   A. 99% of fluorine absorbed from GIT is deposited in calcified tissues
   B. The half life of fluorine in body is 8 years
   C. Changes are more marked in appendicular skeleton than axial skeleton
   D. The skull and tubular bones are spared in osteosclerosis
   E. The posterior longitudinal ligament is spared from calcification

53. Fluorosis:
   A. In all patients there is osteopenia initially which is replaced by osteosclerosis
   B. Extensive osteophyte formation causes spinal stenosis
   C. Periosteal reaction can happen only if there is pathological fracture
   D. Bony excrescence seen in calcaneum
   E. Calcification of interosseus membrane is a characteristic feature

54. Fluorosis:
   A. After cessation of fluoride exposure, all the changes revert to normal except sclerosis
   B. When fluorides are used for treatment of osteoporosis, the changes are same as fluorosis
   C. Genu valgum is a complication of fluorosis
   D. There is no change in medullary cavity in fluorosis
   E. In fluorosis, there is no increase in compressive or tensile strength

55. Associations of osteopoikilosis:
   A. Osteopathia striata
   B. Spinal stenosis
   C. Dystocia
   D. Dwarfism
   E. Dermatofibrosis lenticularis

56. Osteopoikilosis:
   A. No change in the size or number of lesions
   B. Carpal and tarsal bones are spared
   C. Bilaterally symmetrical
   D. Increased uptake in bone scans
   E. Spares the rib
   F. Increased uptake in bone scan

57. Differential diagnosis of osteophytes:
   A. DISH   B. Acromegaly
   C. Psoriasis   D. Alkaptonuria
   E. Inflammatory bowel disease

58. **Differential diagnosis of bony excrescences:**
    A. Hypoparathyroidism
    B. Hyperparathyroidism
    C. Hypophosphatemia
    D. DISH
    E. Fluorosis

59. **Hypophosphatasia—recognized features:**
    A. Wide cranial sutures
    B. Craniostenosis
    C. Diminished urinary excretion of phosphoethanolamine
    D. Diminished metaphyseal calcification
    E. Short 4th metacarpal

60. **Artifical hip prosthesis:**
    A. 1 mm radiolucent lesion at cement bone interface suggests loosening
    B. Periosteal reaction is normal
    C. Exuberant heterotopic bone formation occurs
    D. 25% are hot after one year
    E. Presence of infection is a contraindication for arthrography

61. **Hip prosthesis:**
    A. 95% of prosthesis are successful in ten years
    B. 25% of prosthesis are loose in X-rays after ten years
    C. 10% of hips require revision after ten years
    D. Particle disease increases chance of fracture
    E. Failure from infection of hip prosthesis is low

62. **Hip prosthesis sepsis:**
    A. Good success with debridement if replacement has been recent
    B. Most common infection is Staphylococcus aureus
    C. Dental procedures increase risk
    D. With gram-negative bacteria the reimplantation should be done as soon as possible
    E. Antibiotic laden cement should be given for two stage reimplantation procedure

63. **Hip prosthesis sepsis:**
    A. Involves the femoral side, but not the acetabular side
    B. Sclerosis
    C. Bone destruction
    D. Cortical thickening
    E. Periosteal reaction

64. **Radiological signs and causes:**
    A. Ant eater appearance—talonavicular fusion
    B. C sign—talar coalition
    C. Brim sign—aneurysmal bone cyst
    D. Carpal crowding—rheumatoid arthritis
    E. Tear drop sign—blow out fracture

65. **Radiological signs and causes:**
    A. Sausage digit—psoriasis
    B. Ivory phalanx—Paget's disease
    C. H shaped vertebra—renal failure
    D. Rugger jersey spine—renal failure
    E. Pedestal sign—loosening of hip prosthesis

66. **Radiological signs:**
    A. Presence of half moon sign indicates posterior dislocation of shoulder
    B. Fish vertebra is a feature of sickle cell disease
    C. Trough sign indicates presence of fracture dislocation of shoulder
    D. Signet ring sign is seen in aneurysmal bone cyst
    E. Cockade image—pathognomonic for intraosseus lipoma

67. **Following associations are well recognized:**
    A. Spiculation at metaphysis and phenylketonuria
    B. Periosteal new bone formation along the phalanges of toes in rubella
    C. Thickening of the mandible due to periosteal new bone formation in rubella
    D. Erosion of proximal end of tibia in congenital syphilis
    E. Dense outline of the epiphyses and healing scurvy

68. **Metaphyseal abnormalities occur in:**
    A. Engelmann's disease
    B. Pyle's disease
    C. Ollier's disease
    D. Osteopetrosis
    E. Turner's syndrome

69. **Paget's disease in maxilla and mandible:**
    A. Root absorption
    B. Hypercementosis
    C. Widening of periodontal membrane
    D. Leontiasis ossium
    E. Orange peel appearance in intraoral views

70. **Prosthesis and loosening:**
    A. Diffuse uptake increase in bone scan is seen only in infection and not in loosening
    B. If uptake in gallium scan is less than bone scan, infection is ruled out
    C. Bone scan has an accuracy of 90%.
    D. Labeled WBC scans use labeled lymphocytes
    E. Gallium scan shows increased uptake only in infection and not in loosening

71. **Prosthesis and loosening:**
    A. Gallium scan has a 95% accuracy
    B. PET scanning with FDG is the best method, with highest accuracy
    C. Labelled leucocytes show increased uptake only when there is infection
    D. Antibodies to IgM antibodies are higly specific
    E. Sulfur colloid imaging should be combined with labeled leucocyte scanning for better results

72. **Irradiation is associated with:**
    A. Scoliosis
    B. Osteochondroma
    C. Poor healing of shoulder girdle fractures
    D. Sacroiliitis
    E. Meningiomas

73. **Juvenile scoliosis:**
    A. Females are affected more than males
    B. Radiographs should be taken PA than AP
    C. Worse prognosis than infantile scoliosis
    D. Improved prognosis with earlier presentation
    E. Convex to left side

74. **Loosers zones are seen in:**
    A. Osteoporosis
    B. Neurofibromatosis
    C. Hyperphosphatasia
    D. Hypophosphatasia
    E. Renal tubular dysfunction

75. **Increased uptake in bone scan is seen in the following lesions:**
    A. Vitamin D excess
    B. Fibróus dysplasia
    C. Cerebral infarction
    D. Osteomalacia
    E. Normal breast

76. **Loosers zones:**
    A. Heal with immobilization
    B. Difficult to differentiate with stress fracture
    C. Good callus response
    D. Bilateral and symmetrical
    E. Readily progresses to complete fracture

77. **Common sites of Loosers zones:**
    A. Medial side of scapula
    B. Greater tuberosity
    C. Distal 1/3rd of ulna
    D. Proximal 1/3rd radius
    E. Lateral femoral neck

78. **Bone infarct is seen in:**
    A. Hypopituitarism
    B. Pheochromocytoma
    C. Osteochondroses
    D. Sarcoidosis
    E. Polycythemia rubra vera

79. **Bone infarct:**
    A. No changes are seen unless cortex is involved
    B. Calcification is seen parallel to cotex
    C. Areas of dense bone indicate necrosed bone
    D. Cortical infarction requires occlusion of the nutrient vessels
    E. Cortical infarction is common in children

80. **Complications of bone infarct:**
    A. Coned epiphysis
    B. Fibrosarcoma
    C. Bone cyst
    D. Malignant fibrous histiocytoma
    E. Osteoarthritis

81. **Loss of lamina dura is a recognized feature of:**
    A. Ameloblastoma   B. Hyperparathyroidism
    C. Nasopalatine cyst   D. Dentigerous cyst
    E. Osteoporosis

82. **Pseudohypoparathyroidism:**
    A. X-linked dominant inheritance
    B. Mental status is unaffected
    C. Dentition is delayed
    D. Accelerated skeletal maturation
    E. Multiple exostosis seen in the diaphysis is a feature

83. **Pseudohypoparathyroidism and pseudo-pseudohypoparathyroidism:**
    A. Calcification of basal ganglia is more common in pseudo
    B. Soft tissue calcification is more common in pseudo-pseudo
    C. Metacarpal shortening is more common in pseudo-pseudo
    D. Metatarsal shortening is more common in pseudo
    E. Calcium and phosphorus are normal in pseudo and abnormal in pseudo-pseudo

84. **Acromegaly:**
    A. Frontal sinuses are large
    B. Hyperostosis of inner table
    C. Occipital protuberances are absent
    D. Anterior scalloping of vertebrae
    E. Disk space narrowing

85. **Osteopoikilosis:**
    A. Rare before three years
    B. Autosomal dominant inheritance
    C. Identical to bone islands in histology
    D. Ossification of lamella within haversian systems
    E. Ossification of calcified cartilage rest

86. **Osteopoikilosis:**
    A. In epiphysis, seen in subchondral location
    B. In metaphysis adherent to endosteum
    C. Upto 10 mm
    D. Compact bone
    E. Joint effusion seen

87. **Differential diagnosis of sclerotic lesions mimicking osteopoikilosis:**
    A. Osteopathia striata   B. Mastocytosis
    C. Melorheostosis   D. Tuberous sclerosis
    E. Metastasis

88. **Hypoparathyroidism:**
    A. Seen in 50% of thyroidectomies
    B. Maternal hyperparathyroidism is a well recognised cause
    C. Autoimmune disease is common in males
    D. Thinning of skull due to low parathyroid hormones
    E. Increased osteophyte formation

89. **Hypoparathyroidism:**
    A. Causes hyperdensity in the iliac crest
    B. Produces growth recovery lines
    C. Sacroiliac joint is spared
    D. Calcification spares the anterior longitudinal ligament
    E. Falx is calcified

90. **Joint prosthesis:**
    A. 90% of joint prosthesis are loosened by 10 years
    B. Loosening of prosthesis is an immune reaction
    C. Infection occurs in 10% of prosthesis
    D. Staphylococcus aureus is the most common cause of prosthesis infection
    E. 75% of infection occurs after the first year

91. **Joint prosthesis:**
    A. It is essential to differentiate infection and loosening as treatment is different
    B. ESR and CRP are specific for infection and not elevated in loosening
    C. A periprosthetic uptake equal to the surrounding bone is considered normal
    D. Focal uptake at the tip of cemented prosthesis after one year is indicative of infection
    E. Any increased uptake after one year, in a porous prosthesis, is abnormal

92. **Pathological fracture occurs in:**
    A. Acromegaly
    B. Hyperparathyroidism
    C. Hemodialysis
    D. Spinal bifida
    E. Paget's disease

93. **Paget's disease:**
    A. Biopsy is avoided during the lytic phase of the Paget's disease
    B. Progression is always sequential from 1 through 3rd stages
    C. Monostotic in 25% of instances
    D. Pelvis is involved in 2/3rd of cases
    E. MRI shows high signal in the first phase, which enhances on contrast.

94. **Features of rickets with normal vitamin D and phosphate metabolism:**
    A. Fanconi's syndrome
    B. Hypophosphatasia
    C. Hepatitis/Cirrhosis
    D. Axial osteomalacia
    E. Schmidt's metaphyseal dysplasia

ANSWERS

1. **A-F, B-T, C-F, D-F, E-F**
Fractures of hips are more important and serious as ther is 20% mortality and 20% require long-term care. X-ray is not very sensitive and there must be atleast 35% reduction in bone density to be detected by X-rays. The incidence of osteoporotic fractures is expected to rise due to increased life expectancy.

2. **A-T, B-T, C-T, D-T, E-F**
DXA—X-rays emitted from X-ray tube used to provide X-ray beam with relative energies of 40 and 70 keV.

3. **A-F, B-T, C-F, D-T, E-F**
This is a self limiting disease. It is more common in the left side. Males in the middle age group are commonly affected. There is rapid development of pain and swelling around joint.

4. **A-F, B-F, C-F, D-F, E-F**
Joint space narrowing and collapse of bone are not seen. Pathological fracture can be seen. The bone scan is very hot, without any cold areas. Bone scan is the most sensitive.
MRI shows diffuse bone marrow oedema in the femoral head and neck.

5. **A-F, B-T, C-T, D-F, E-T**
Joint space narrowing and bone destruction are not seen. Low signal in T2 and high signal in T2 are features of bone marrow edema. The same symptoms will be repeated in another joint after a period of 6-9 months. Knee, ankle, hip are affected, Transient, migrates to adjacent joints.

6. **A-F, B-F, C-F, D-F, E-F**
Almost all the foreign bodies are echogenic in ultrasound. Ultrasound is superior for non-radiopaque foreign bodies in soft tissue. Hypoechoic rim is seen due to inflammatory response around the foreign body and is normally seen after 24 hours. Posterior shadowing does not depend on the composition, but on the surface of the foreign body. A flat, smooth surface produces dirty reverberation shadows. Irregular, small curvature, produce clean shadowing. Some foreign bodies can produce both.

7. **A-T, B-F, C-T, D-F, E-T**
The tarsal tunnel is situated in the plantar aspect of the foot and extends from the posteromedial side of the ankle to the plantar aspect of foot. There are two components, the upper and lower tarsal tunnel . The upper tibiotalar tunnel is covered by aponeurosis and has flexor digitorum longus, flexor hallucis longus, tibialis

posterior and posterior tibial neurovascular bundle. The lower talocalcenal part, is covered by flexor retinaculum and has posterior tibial nerve.

8. **A-F, B-F, C-F, D-F, E-F**
Neuropathic changes are most common in the intertarsal and tarsometatarsal joints. Septic arthritis is most common in the MTP joints. Ulcers are common under the first and fifth metatarsal head. Although predominantly neuropathic joint is painless, pain can be seen in the acute stages. The MRI findings of neuropathic joints, osteomyelitis, septic arthritis and inflammation are similar and cannot be distinguished based on signal characteristics. They are low in T1, high in T2 and show enhancement. Increased incidence of Lisfranc's dislocation is also seen in the diabetics.

9. **A-T, B-T, C-F, D-F, E-F**
Presence of ulcer, sinus tract, cortical interruption, abscesses favour osteomyelitis. Increased density, destruction, fragmentation, debri, dislocation are more common in neuropathic joints.

10. **A-F, B-T, C-F, D-T, E-F**
Tophi have intermediate signal in T1 and low signal in T2 and do enhance on contrast. Trauma, infection, RA are other causes of bursitis. Granulomatous reaction does not happen in gout and is usually a response to foreign bodies or granulomatous infection. Gout also seen in ear and kidneys.

11. **A-F, B-T, C-T, D-T, E-T**
Hypercalcemia—Hyperparathyroidism, Lung carcinoma, breast cancer, sarcoidosis, berylliosis, TB, leprosy coccidioidomycosis, histoplasmosis, iatrogenic, bone metastasis, multiple myeloma, hematologic malignancy, other malignancies, drugs (thiazide, antacids), hypervitaminosis D and A, milk-alkali syndrome, familial immobilisation MEN, Addison's, pheochromocytoma, hyperthyroidism, AIDS, chronic liver disease.

12. **A-F, B-T, C-T, D-F, E-F**
Pancreatitis causes hypocalcemia due to endotoxemia.

13. **A-T, B-F, C-T, D-F, E-T**
80% of patients have skull and spine lesions. Bone scans cannot differentiate Paget's and metastasis. Fibrosarcoma is the second most common malignancy in Paget's. Serum calcium and phosphorus are normal in Paget's. Calcium can be high in immobilisation. Hypercalciuria of bone lysis produces renal stones.

14. **A-F, B-T, C-T, D-T, E-T**
Other causes are steroids, NSAIDs, Immunosuppressants, trauma, radiation, burns, RA, SLE, scleroderma, pancreatitis, fat embolism,

septic arthritis, pregnancy, DM, gout, hyperlipidemia, sickle cell, Gaucher's, polycythemia, Caissons disease, arteritis.

15. **A-F, B-F, C-T, D-F, E-F**
Hyperparathyroidism causes high calcium and alkaline phosphatase. Hypoparathyroidism causes decreased calcium.
Myeloma—high calcium, normal alkaline phosphatase, Paget's, Calcium—Normal, High—Phosphatase

16. **A-T, B-F, C-T, D-F, E-F**
Hypophosphatasia—low alkaline phosphatase and defective bone mineralisation. Can be autosomal recessive/dominant. High pyridoxal 5 phosphate. Perinatal type lethal absent mineralisation. Rachitic changes fractures, spurs; infantile—mild open fontanelle, craniosynostosis, Childhood milder, Rachitic, lucencies from metaphysis to epiphysis; adults – pseudofractures in lateral aspect of femur, stress fractures.

17. **A-T, B-F, C-T, D-F, E-T**
1% incidence of sarcomatous change. Paraplegia is caused by vertebral body fracture and cord compression. Calcium is elevated but phosphate is normal. Alkaline phosphatase is elevated. Vertebral collapse can cause paraplegia.

18. **A-F, B-T, C-F, D-T, E-T**
High signal is usually not seen in the intertrochanteric region. Recovery takes 2-6 months. Metastasis, arthritis, sympathetic dystrophy, disuse atrophy, PVNS and synovial chondromatosis are other differential diagnosis.

19. **A-T, B-F, C-F, D-F, E-T**
Presents with pain, swelling and limited range of movements. Common in the lower limb.
Osteoporosis seen in 3-6 weeks after onset. Involves both the cortical and cancellous bone.

20. **A-T, B-F, C-T, D-F, E-F**
Sarcomatous change is seen, but not very common. Biconcave vertebra is a common feature in osteoporosis. Axial skeletan and prox femur affected. Seen after 40 years, 50-70 years, more common in men.

21. **A-F, B-T, C-F, D-F, E-T**
Cord compression common due to platybasia. Conductive sensorineural hearing loss is seen. Vision can be affected due to compression of optic nerve.

22. **A-F, B-T, C-F, D-F, E-F**
Incremental fractures are seen in the lateral side of the neck of the femur. Osteoporosis circumscripta frontal, occipital bones, calcium is normal. Hydroxyproline level increased in urine and serum.

23. **A-F, B-T, C-T, D-F, E-F**
The skull is enlarged with frontal bossing and dilated superficial cranial muscles. Leonine facies due to facial involvement. High output cardiac failure soon.

24. **A-T, B-F, C-F, D-F, E-T**
Histiocytosis—Hand-Schüller-Christian disease—DI, exophthalmos, histiocytosis, urticaria
Sarcoidosis—Lupus prenio, erythema, bony changes

25. **A-T, B-T, C-T, D-T, E-T**
Renal failure, radiation, SLE, rheumatoid arthritis, polyarteritis nodosa, dialysis, thermal injury, tumours, Cushing's, alcoholism are other recognised causes. Sickle is the commonest hemoglobinopathy.

26. **A-T, B-F, C-F, D-T, E-T**
And medial femoral condyle, capitellum.

27. **A-T, B-T, C-F, D-F, E-T**
Repeated trauma is the common cause of lunate avascular necrosis in manual labourers. Develops 9-19 months after renal transplantation. Common in the shoulder and is related to the original renal disease.

28. **A-F, B-T, C-F, D-T, E-F**
Bilateral knee involvement is seen in 1/3 rd of cases. The fragment can grow or resorb or calcify. Osteochondritis dissecans common in talus.

29. **A-T, B-T, C-T, D-F, E-T**
60-70% of avascular necrosis of femoral head is due to femoral neck fracture, 15-25% is due to hip dislocation and 10% is due to slipped femoral epiphyses.
The joint space is not narrowed in avascular necrosis. Unless there is degenerative disease.

30. **A-F, B-T, C-T, D-F, E-F**
Sagittal images are the optimal. In advanced stages, contrast enhancement is seen at interface. The fracture cleft is usually hypointense, but a hyperintense band can be seen due to edema or articular fluid. Inhomogenous edema is seen.

31. **A-T, B-T, C-T, D-T, E-T**
    Perthes' disease is the most common cause. Meyer's dysplasia is the most common differential diagnosis, but this occurs at 2 years,(earlier the Perthes'), mild or absent clinical symptoms, retarded skeletal maturation, and can be unilateral or bilateral. Sclerosis and metaphyseal collapse are not seen. Other differential diagnosis include hypothyroidism, epiphyseal dysplasia, infection and eosinophilic granuloma.

32. **A-T, B-T, C-T, D-T, E-F**
    Recurrence is believed to be due to persistence of ununited fragment and fragmentation of femoral head weakened by revascularization. Large femoral head is called coxa magna. Coxa plana, degenerative joint disease, osteochondroma like lesions. A common complication is the saggying rope sign, which is a dense curved line in the metaphysis, in the suprolateral aspect of head, which is a shadow caused by anterior or lateral edge of severely deformed femoral head.

33. **A-F, B-F, C-T, D-T, E-T**
    Lateral III and IV stages, females, delayed diagnosis, increased age at onset, extensive metaphyseal or epiphyseal involvement, lateral displacement of femoral head.

34. **A-T, B-F, C-F, D-F, E-T**

A	high	int	fat
B	high	high	blood
C	low	high	fluid
D	low	low	fibrous

    0—normal
    I—normal X-ray. Abnormal bone scan/MRI
    IIA—sclerosis, osteopenia
    IIB—+ crescent sign
    IIIA—crescent sign, cyst
    IIIB—altered femoral contour, subchondral fracture
    IV—marked collapse of femoral head, acetabular involvement
    V—joint space narrowing

35. **A-F, B-T, C-T, D-F, E-T**
    Kienböck's disease is osteonecrosis of lunate bone. Mechanical factors are a predisposing cause. In negative ulnar variance, the ulna is situated proximal to the radius, and it puts mechanical force on lunate. Common in the right hand. Often managed by surgical methods including vascular bone grafting and arthrodesis.

36. **A-F, B-T, C-F, D-F, E-T**
    I—X-ray normal. MRI low signal in T1, subtle fracture in CT
    II—sclerosed lunate, flattened lateral border
    III—collapsed lunate, proximal migration of capitate, instability
    IV—degenerative changes in lunate, mid carpal, radiocarpal joints.

37. **A-F, B-T, C-T, D-T, E-T**

38. **A-T, B-T, C-T, D-T, E-T**
    Steroid injection, loose bodies and trauma, vascular insufficiency
    are supposed to be causative factors for spontaneous osteonecrosis
    of knee. Meniscal injury is associated in 80% and steroid injection
    in 50%.

39. **A-F, B-T, C-F, D-T, E-T**
    It is commonly seen in the seventh decade. Commonly seen in the
    weight bearing medial condyle. Only in 5% it involves the femoral
    condyle and only rarely the tibial plateau is affected. Medial
    Femoral condyle is flattened. Bone scan is the most sensitive
    method.
    X-ray changes take 3 months. Subcondral fracture is seen in 6-9
    months.

40. **A-F, B-T, C-T, D-F, E-F**
    Osteomalacia—lack of calcium and phosphorus for mineralisation.
    Renal osteodystrophy, hyperthyroidism, neurofibroma, fibrosis
    dysplasia anticonvulsants, gastric surgeries, small bowel mal-
    absorption syndromes, phosphates, phytic acids are other causes.

41. **A-F, B-F, C-T, D-F, E-F**
    Myositis ossificans progressiva.

42. **A-T, B-F, C-T, D-T, E-T**

43. **A-T, B-T, C-T, D-T, E-F**
    Brachycephaly, delayed dentition, large sella and delayed closure
    of fontanelles are other features in the skull. Delayed maturation,
    osteoporosis, fragmented epiphysis are also seen.

44. **A-T, B-T, C-T, D-F, E-F**

45. **A-F, B-T, C-T, D-F, E-F**
    Thyroid acropachy seen after treatment of hyperthyroidism; M=F,
    Exophthalmos, pretibial myxedema, periostitis seen. Affects
    diaphysis of small tubular bones feathery periosteal reaction. Soft
    tissue swelling seen, occasionally long bones affected. Seen after
    thyroidectomy for thyrotoxicosis—probably secondary to exposure
    to LATS.

46. **A-F, B-T, C-T, D-T, E-F**
    Periosteal reaction is characteristic in the diaphyseal region and is usually bilaterally symmetrical, lacy or solid or spiculated. Erosions are not characteristic.

47. **A-F, B-T, C-F, D-F, E-T**
    Small stature, slender bones and small pituitary fossa are other features. Delayed appearance and closure of epiphysis and osteopenia are seen.

48. **A-T, B-T, C-T, D-F, E-T**
    Thymus is enlarged. Osteoporosis, cortical tunelling fractures, periostitis, wedged vertebrae are other feature.

49. **A-T, B-F, C-T, D-F, E-T**
    Heart failure, pleural effusion and ascites are other features.

50. **A-T, B-T, C-F, D-F, E-T**
    Callus formation is exuberant in Cushing's syndrome. Avascular necrosis and premature osteoarthritis are other features.

51. **A-T, B-T, C-F, D-T, E-F**
    <1 ppm—normal, >2 ppm—dental mottling, >4 ppm—skeletal fluorosis, >8 ppm—osteosclerosis, >10 ppm—growth disturbance.

52. **A-F, B-T, C-F, D-T, E-F**
    50% of fluorine absorbed from the GIT is excreted in urine. Of the 50% that is retained, 99% is deposited in calcified tissues. The changes are more marked in axial skeleton. Calcification is seen in paraspinal, intraspinal, sacrotuberous, iliolumbar ligaments.

53. **A-F, B-T, C-F, D-T, E-T**
    The typical findings in fluorosis are osteosclerosis, ligamental calcification, periostitis, osteophytes and osseous excrescences. In all patients osteosclerosis is the initial feature and only in a few, osteopenia is the initial feature. Extensive periosteal reaction, is seen bilaterally. Bony excrescences are also seen in tibial tuberosity, proximal humerus and posterior surface of femur.

54. **A-F, B-F, C-T, D-F, E-F**
    After cessation of fluoride exposure, the osteosclerosis reverts to normal, but with coarsening of trabeculae. The other changes are not reversed. When fluorides are used in treatment of osteoporosis, the changes are similar to fluorosis but ligamental calcification is absent. The cortex is thickened and medullary cavity is narrowed in fluorosis. There is increase in compressive strength but decrease in tensile strength. The elasticity is also decreased and the incidence of fracture is increased. Even when fluorine is used for osteoporosis, there is no increase in strength of bone.

55. A-T, B-T, C-T, D-T, E-T
Osteopathia striata and melorheostosis have probably the same etiology. A combination of 3 is called mixed sclerosing bone dystrophy.
25% have cutaneous lesion called dermatofibrosis lenticularis disseminata, which is whitish (Buschke-Ollendorff syndrome).

56. A-F, B-F, C-T, D-F, E-T, F-F
The lesions are well-defined 3-10 mm, uniform size in the metaphysis and epiphysis. Can increase or decrease in size.
Common in carpal and tarsal bones, pelvis and scapula. Occasionally lumbosacral spine. No increased uptake—condensation of spongiosa.
Ribs, clavicle, skull are spared.

57. A-T, B-T, C-T, D-T, E-T
Degenerative disease, fluorosis, Reiter's disease, neuropathic disease are other causes

58. A-T, B-F, C-T, D-T, E-T
Also seen in plasma cell dyscrasia.

59. A-T, B-T, C-F, D-T, E-F
Hypophosphatasia—other features—Bowel legs, craniosynostosis, undermineralised skull wide metaphysis delayed closure of fontanelles, metaphyseal dysplasia, fractures, Beady ribs, funnel chart, short stature, osteomalacia, premature loss of teeth and wide metaphysis. Urine phosphoethanolamine is elevated. Short 4th metacarpal in turner's pseudohypoparathroidism, infection, trauma.

60. A-F, B-F, C-T, D-F, E-T
Lucent bone at cement bone interface > 2mm, wide cement bone lucent zone, migration of components cement fracture, periosteal reaction, movement of components on stress indicate loosening or infection. Hot spot is very variable and is considered normal upto one year.

61. A-F, B-F, C-F, D-T, E-F
Particle disease extensive lysis around prosthesis (polyethylene), near tipt of femoral component or medial border due to giant cell response. Cement disease seen in cemented polymethylmethacrylate prosthesis heterotopic bone formation, dislocation acetabular wear are other complication 1.3% infection, require revision arthroplasty 50% develop loosening by one year, 30% require revision, 1/3rd of infection occurs before 3 months, 1/3rd 3 months, 1 year, 1/3rd after one year.

62. **A-T, B-F, C-T, D-F, E-F**

Staph. epidermidis is the most common organism followed by Staph. aureus. In dental procedures Strep. viridans is the organism. Patient presents with pain at rest and activity, with high ESR and fever. In proper patients, patients can be managed by only debridement AND IV antibiotics. One stage reimplantation, requires antibiotic laden cement. Two stage reimplantation uses revision prosthesis, without need for antibiotic cement. In infection with gram-negative bacteria, reimplantation requires 12 months. In other less virulent organisms, reimplantation can be done in three months.

63. **A-F, B-T, C-T, D-T, E-T**

Both sides of the joint are affected.

64. **A-F, B-T, C-F, D-F, E-T**

An ant eater appearance is seen in calcaneonavicular fusion. This is caused by the lateral film of the foot, which shows a tubular projection from the anterior margin of the calcaneum, which is the bony bar extending to the navicular bone. C sign is seen in lateral film of the foot and is the bony ridge between talus and sustentaculum tali. Brim sign is seen in Paget's disease of the pelvis, when there is thickening and sclerosis of the ileopectinate line in the pelvic brim. Carpal crowding is when the two rows of carpal bones overlap and this is seen in volar perilunate dislocation. Tear drop sign is a tear drop shaped projection seen from the orbital floor due to fracture and herniation of orbital contents, fat and inferior rectus muscle.

65. **A-T, B-F, C-F, D-T, E-T**

Sausage digit refer to soft tissue swelling of a single digit, which is very common in psoriasis. Ivory phalanx, refers to sclerosis of a single phalanx and is also typically seen in psoriasis. Ivory vertebra is seen in Paget's disease. Rugger jersey spine refers to the appearance of secondary hyperparathyroidism, which shows osteopenia with end plate sclerosis. Pedestal sign is due to two opaque lines projecting from the tip of femoral component of a hip prosthesis and indicates looseing. H shaped vertebra is typically seen in sickle cell disease.

66. **A-F, B-F, C-T, D-F, E-T**

Half moon sign refers to partial overlap of the medial aspect of humeral head over the glenoid rim. If this is lost, it indicates posterior dislocation of shoulder. Trough sign refers to visualization of two cortical margins in the head of the humerus. The inner line is the normal medial cortex of head of humerus. The lateral one is due to impacted fracture caused when the posterior and internally rotated humerus impacts against the anterior glenoid rim. Signet ring sign refers to a ring shaped appearance of scaphoid seen due to rotatory subluxation. Cockade image refers to the typical lytic lesion with calcification seen in the calcaneal intraosseous lipoma.

67. **A-T, B-F, C-F, D-T, E-T**

68. **A-F, B-T, C-T, D-T, E-F**
Engelmann's disease is a type of diaphyseal dysplasia. Pyles is a craniometaphyseal dysplasia. Ollier's disease is multiple enchondromas with dysplastic metaphysis. Osteopetrosis—Metaphyseal bands, sclerosis.

69. **A-T, B-T, C-T, D-T, E-F**
Bones are expanded with thic trabeculae.

70. **A-F, B-T, C-F, D-F, E-F**
Define uptake can be normal/infection/loosening, focal uptake at tip of cement—loosening. Bone scan accuracy 50-70%, if gallium scan is normal less uptake than abnormal bone scan—no infection labeled neutrophils are used since they are absent in loosening and present in infection gallium detechts inflammation and positive in both.

71. **A-F, B-F, C-F, D-T, E-T**
Bone scan—60% accurate, uptake depends on bone formation and vascularity, diffuse uptake normal for one year and more if porous prosthesis, increased uptake in both infection and loosening, not specific. Gallium scan—80% accurate, uptake depends on inflammation and infection, increased uptake in both, but more in infection, uptake more than bone scan indicates infection, less than bone scan indicates loosening.
Labeled leucocytes—90% accurate, labeled neutrophils, hence uptake only by infection and not loosening which has predominantly histiocytic infiltrate, only confusion is with uptake in normal marrow, compared with bone marrow imaging with sulfur colloid. FDG—PET-increased uptake in both, as good as gallium, not better.

72. **A-T, B-T, C-T, D-T, E-T**

73. **A-T, B-T, C-T, D-T, E-T**
Juvenile scoliosis 4-10 years, females more common, 70% progress, hence surgery required unlike infantile scoliosis which can correct spontaneously common in dorsolumbar region. PA view reduce radiation to breast.

74. **A-F, B-T, C-T, D-T, E-T**
Osteomalacia is the most common cause.
Renal disease, osteogenesis imperfecta, hyperthyroidism, X-linked, hypophosphatemia fibrous dysplasia, Paget's disease, rickets and vitamin D malabsorption are other causes.

75. **A-T, B-T, C-T, D-T, E-T**

76. **A-T, B-T, C-F, D-T, E-T**
Callus formation is either absent or little.

77. **A-F, B-F, C-F, D-F, E-F**
Lateral side of scapula, lesser trochanter, proximal 1/3rd ulna, distal 1/3rd radius, medial femoral neck, greater trochanter, ischiopubic rami, ischial tuberosity, phalanges and metatarsals.

78. **A-T, B-T, C-T, D-T, E-T**
The same causes as avascular necrosis.

79. **A-T, B-T, C-F, D-F, E-T**
X-ray changes are seen only after the cortex is involved. In acute stage there is lucency, but in chronic change the lesion is rimmed by dense serpiginous calcification or ossification, parallel to cortex. Areas of dense bone indicate revascularisation.
Cortical infarction requires occlusion of nutrient and periosteal vessels and hence common in children, where the periosteum is loosely attached and easily elevated.

80. **A-T, B-T, C-T, D-T, E-T**
Malignant conversion is a recognised complication. Epiphyseal abnormalities are also commonly seen.

81. **A-T, D-T, C-F, D-T, E-T**
Metabolic—hyperparathyroidism, osteomalacia, fibrous dysplasia, Endocrine—osteoporosis, Cushing's, Neoplastic—histiocytosis, Cementoma, ameloblastoma, metastasis, myeloma, leukemia Infections, Paget's, scleroderma

82. **A-T, B-F, C-T, D-T, E-T**
Affected patients are usually mentally retarded. Dentition is delayed or hypoplastic and caries are associated. Shortening of metacarpals and metatarsals especially 4th, 5th and 1st. Accelerated skeletal maturation leads to dwarfism. Calcification is seen in basal ganglia and soft tissue.

83. **A-T, B-F, C-T, D-F, E-F**
Calcification in soft tissue and basal ganglia and metacarpal and metatarsal shortening are salient features of pseudo and

pseudo-pseudohypothyroidism. Basal ganglia and soft tissue calcification are more common in pseudohypoparathyroidism. Metacarpal and metatarsal shortening are more common in pseudo-pseudohypoparathyroidism. Calcium and phosphorus are normal in pseudo-pseudohypoparathyroidism. In pseudohypoparathyroidism, calcium is low and phosphorus is high. In pseudo-pseudo there is normal response to PTH injection. In pseudo, there is resistance to PTH injection.

84. **A-T, B-T, C-F, D-F, E-T**
Occipital protuberances are large. Posterior scalloping is seen, not anterior. Osteophytes are also seen. Disk space is narrowed due to degeneration. Premature osteoarthritis is a common feature.

85. **A-T, B-T, C-T, D-T, E-F**
It can be seen in any age, but rare before three years. It is sporadic or autosomal dominant inherited. It has osteoblasts, osteoclasts and osteocytes, but no calcified cartilage matrix, suggestive that is not derived from ossification of cartilage rest.

86. **A-F, B-T, C-T, D-T, E-T**
Characteristic location is eccentric in metaphysis, adherent to endosteum. In epiphysis does not abut subchondral bone. 3-10 mm, islands of compact bone. Joint effusion and pain is seen in 25%.

87. **A-F, B-T, C-F, D-T, E-T**
Mastocytosis, tuberous scleoris and metastasis are not uniform/ symmetrical/localised in metaphysis and epiphysis. Metastases affects the axial skeleton unlike osteopoikilosis and increased uptake can be seen.

88. **A-F, B-T, C-F, D-F, E-T**
Seen in less than 15% of thyroidectomies. Maternal hyperparathyroidism means high calcium into the fetal calcification which by feedback suppresses the parathyroid in the fetus. Autoimmune disease is common in females. The skull vault is thickened.

89. **A-T, B-T, C-T, D-F, E-T**
The common features are skull thickening, calcification of falx and basal ganglia, subcutaneous calcification, spinal ossification, premature fusion of epiphysis, osteosclerosis and hypoplastic dentition. Soft tissue calcification is common around the hips, shoulders, and can be painful if there is calcific periarthritis. Ligamental calcification affects all the ligaments, including the anterior longitudinal ligaments.Enthesopathy is seen but with sparing of the sacroiliac joints.

90. **A-F, B-T, C-F, D-F, E-F**

Only 50% of prosthesis are loosened by 10 years. Loosening is believed to be an inflammatory immune response. The cement fragments elicit inflammatory response, bringing phagocytes and other mediators, which are progressively augmented, resulting in the loosening of the prosthesis bone interface. One-third of infection occurs in the first three months, one-third before one year and one-third after one year. Infection 0.5-3%.

91. **A-T, B-F, C-T, D-F, E-F**

Loosening is managed by single stage revision arthroplasty. Infection requires removal or prosthesis, treatment of infection and then revision arthroplasty. ESR and CRP can be elevated in both. Diffuse increase in uptake can be normal for one year in cemented prosthesis, and for longer duration in porous prosthesis as it produces more new bone formation. Hence, increased uptake after one year in cemented prosthesis is abnormal and can represent infection or loosening. A focal uptake at the tip of a cemented prosthesis is a typical finding of loosening and not infection.

92. **A-F, B-T, C-T, D-F, E-T**

93. **A-T, B-F, C-T, D-T, E-T**

The four stages are I—lytic, II—mixed, III— sclerotic, IV— malignant phase. The progression is not necessarily sequential and sclerotic can be the first manifestation. More than 3/4th of the cases are polyostotic.

94. **A-F, B-T, C-F, D-T, E-T**

Only there 3 conditions produce rachitic changes with normal Vitamin D phosphorus metabolism.

High alkaline phosphatase seen in Paget's, osteomalacia, rickets, metastasis, hyperparathyroidism infection, liver pathologies. Low alkaline phosphatase celiac disease, scurvy hypocalcemia seen in hypoparathyroidism, pseudohypoparathyroidism, Vitamin D deficiency and resistant rickets, pancreatitis, hyperphosphatemia, idiopathic, malabsorption.

5

Musculoskeletal Trauma

1. **Trauma:**
   A. Bohler's angle greater than 20 degrees indicates fractured calcaneum
   B. Fracture of the base of the 5th metatarsal is transverse rather than longitudinal
   C. Subcapital femoral neck fracture is unusual in osteoarthritis
   D. Genu valgum predisposes to lateral dislocation of patella
   E. In the knee joint, dislocation at the tibiofemoral joint is more often seen than patellofemoral joint

2. **Classic signs of flexion injury of the cervical spine:**
   A. Neural arch fractures
   B. Pillar and articular process fractures
   C. Widening of interspinous space
   D. Widening of the disc space
   E. Facet joint locking

3. **Instability in a patient with cervical spinal trauma:**
   A. Subluxation more than 4 mm
   B. Angulation more than 15 degrees with associated disc space abnormality
   C. Retropharyngeal space more than 15 mm
   D. Vertebral body compression more than 25% of normal height
   E. Increased interspinous distance

4. **Clavicle fractures and dislocations:**
   A. The lateral third of the clavicle is the most common site to fracture
   B. In fracture of the lateral third, the lateral fragment is usually placed higher than the medial fragment
   C. Pneumothorax is a complication of fractures of medial third of clavicle
   D. Most common bone to be fractured in breech delivery
   E. A complication of central venous line insertion

5. **Clavicular dislocation:**
   A. Sternoclavicular dislocation is more common than acromio-clavicular dislocation
   B. Fracture of the medial third implies severe injury
   C. Sternoclavicular dislocation injures phrenic nerve
   D. Type I acromioclavicular dislocation can be diagnosed only in stress views
   E. The distance between the coracoid and clavicle is unaffected in type III acromioclavicular dislocation

6. **The following are highly unstable fractures:**
   A. Hangman's fracture
   B. Type I odontoid fractures
   C. Unilateral locked facets
   D. Jefferson's fracture
   E. Burst fractures

7. **Fat pad sign in elbow is seen in:**
   A. Intra-articular fracture
   B. Leukemia
   C. Synovial osteochondromatosis
   D. Gout
   E. Neuropathic osteoarthropathy

8. **Eponymous fractures:**
   A. Maisonneuve's—lateral malleolus and proximal fibular shaft
   B. Jone's—proximal 5th metacarpal shaft
   C. Chauffeur's—radial styloid
   D. Bennett—base of 1st metacarpal
   E. Segond—avulsion of lateral margin of tibial plateau

9. **Eponymous fractures:**
   A. Lisfranc—avulsion at medial base of second metatarsal
   B. Boxer's—4th or 5th metacarpal neck
   C. Chance—upper lumbar vertebrae
   D. Monteggia—proximal radial shaft
   E. Galeazzi—distal ulnar shaft

10. **Fractures:**
    A. Barton facture—reversed Colle's fractures
    B. Hutchinson fracture—radial styloid
    C. Smith—dorsal displacement of distal fragment
    D. Game keepers thumb—disruption of radial collateral ligament of thumb
    E. Chopart—mid tarsal joint

11. **Fracture of the talus:**
    A. Associated with avascular necrosis
    B. Usually involves the joint
    C. Associated with fractures of fifth metatarsal
    D. Fracture of talus alters the Bohler's angle
    E. Blood supply to talar dome enters through the proximal talus

12. **Fractures foot:**
    A. Stress fractures commonly involve the fourth and fifth metatarsals
    B. There is increased incidence of Lisfranc's dislocation in diabetes
    C. In Lisfranc's dislocation, the dislocation always occurs in only one direction
    D. Fracture of 2nd metatarsal is usually present in almost all cases of Lisfranc's dislocation
    E. Periosteal reaction can be the only manifestation of stress fracture

13. **Lower limb ossification:**
    A. The femoral head ossifies at 6 months
    B. The greater trochanter ossifies at puberty
    C. The femoral centers fuse with shaft at 20 years
    D. Distal femoral epiphysis begins to ossify at 2 years
    E. The lesser trochanter ossifies at four years

14. **Fractures:**
    A. In AP view of foot, if the medial border of the 2nd metatarsal is aligned with the medial border of the intermediate cuneiform, there is a homolateral dislocation
    B. Freiberg's infraction is common in the fifth metatarsal head
    C. Avulsion fracture at the base of the fifth metatarsal is due to peroneus tertitus muscle
    D. Talar dome avulsion is due to extensor hallucis longus muscle
    E. Mortise view of ankle is performed with external rotation

15. **Normal uptake in gallium scans seen in:**
    A. Salivary glands   B. Stomach mucosa
    C. Epiphyseal plates   D. Nasopharyngeal mucosa
    E. Lymphangiography

16. **Ottawa rules for X-ray of ankle:**
    A. Pain on weight bearing
    B. Tenderness in tip of lateral malleolus
    C. Tenderness in tip of medial malleolus
    D. Pain, but no tenderness
    E. Limitation of ankle movement

17. **Hip fractures and dislocations:**
    A. Fractures of the lesser trochanter are common than those of greater trochanter
    B. Isolated fracture of the lesser trochanter is likely to be metastatic in elderly
    C. Subtrochanteric fractures are more often secondary than primary
    D. Scintigraphy is positive in 5 hours after injury and is done with negative X-rays and positive clinical suspicion
    E. Impacted femoral neck fractures produce more avascular necrosis than non-impacted

18. **Fractures:**
    A. Avascular necrosis is more in intertrochanteric fracture than in subcapital fracture
    B. Anterior dislocations are common than posterior dislocations
    C. Acetabular fractures require CT scan for satisfactory evaluation
    D. Mallet finger is due to disruption of the extensor tendon and is associated with volar plate fractures
    E. Volar plate avulsion fractures are associated with flexion deformity

19. **Stress fractures:**
    A. By definition, occurs only when there is abnormal stress
    B. MRI is more specific than bone scan
    C. Upper limb bones are more commonly affected than lower limb fractures
    D. Shin splints are stress fracture of the tibia
    E. Stress fractures show low signal surrounded by high signal, in both T1 and T2

20. **Hand:**
    A. The most common fracture fragment seen in the dorsal aspect of wrist in lateral film, is a hamate hook fracture
    B. Triquetral bone avulses at the site of attachment of the dorsal radiocarpal ligament
    C. A scapolunate distance more than 1 mm is abnormal
    D. Lunate dislocates posteriorly
    E. Foreshortening of lunate bone in AP film is normal in 50% of individuals

21. **Ottawa rules for X-ray of foot fracture:**
    A. Tender 5th metatarsal   B. Tender talus
    C. Tender navicular   D. Limitation of dorsiflexion
    E. Tender calcaneum

22. **Fractures of hand:**
    A. Bennett's fracture is intra-articular
    B. Rolando's fracture is an impacted fracture of 1st metacarpal
    C. Boxer's fractures are angulated dorsally
    D. Game-Keper's thumb is due to disruption of radial collateral ligament
    E. For diagnosing Skier's thumb, a routine AP view of the hand is enough

23. **Ottawa rules advocate knee X-ray for:**
    A. Over 55 years
    B. Tender patella
    C. Inability to flex the knee to 90 degrees
    D. Tenderness of fibula
    E. Tenderness of medial tibial condyle

24. **Associations of elbow fractures:**
    A. Monteggia's fracture—injury to musculocutaneous nerve
    B. Fractured coronoid—posterolateral dislocation
    C. Supracondylar fractures—involve joints in adults more than kids
    D. Galeazzi's fracture—radial head dislocation
    E. Comparison with other side is unnecessary in children

25. **Metaphyseal fractures are features of:**
    A. Non-accidental injury
    B. Menke's disease
    C. Wilson's disease
    D. Osteogenesis imperfecta
    E. Leukemia

26. **Fractures:**
    A. Pathological fractures are oriented transversely in long bones
    B. Looser's transformation zone are complete fractures seen in osteomalacia
    C. Fracture line is often seen in stress fractures
    D. Suble periosteal reaction is seen in stress fracture at time of presentation
    E. MRI is positive in stress fracture at time of presentation

27. **Sudeck's atrophy:**
    A. Less painful if immobilised in a sling
    B. May be caused by cervical osteoarthritis
    C. Endosteal resorption of bone occurs
    D. Commonly affects multiple joints
    E. May follow myocardial infarction

28. **Sudeck's atrophy:**
    A. Associated with hemiplegia
    B. Associated with frostbite
    C. Diminished flow in bone scan excludes the disease
    D. Delayed images do not show increased uptake in majority
    E. Osteopenia takes atleast 3 months to develop

29. **Avulsion fractures and the muscles involved:**
    A. Anterior superior iliac spine—rectus femoris
    B. Anterior inferior iliac spine—sartorius and tensor fascia lata
    C. Iliac crest—gluteus
    D. Greater trochanter—psoas
    E. Symphysis pubis—adductor muscles

30. **Mandible:**
    A. Midline fracture is part of Le Fort complex
    B. Hypoplasia is associated with juvenile rheumatoid arthritis
    C. Most common place to fracture is coronoid process
    D. Common site of metastasis

31. **Pedicolaminar fractures:**
    A. There are three types
    B. Vertebral comminution is seen in type V
    C. Bilateral changes in type IV
    D. II-narrowed intervertebral disc space
    E. Type IV is the most common combined injury of cervical spine

32. **Pedicolaminar fractures:**
    A. Type IV is caused by hyperextension and compression force on head
    B. Type IV is stable
    C. Interfacetal joint spaces seen in AP film
    D. Lack of superimposition of posterior margins of articular masses at same levels
    E. Rotation of vertebra at the involved level, but not above and below

33. **Posterior dislocation of shoulder:**
    A. Most common type of shoulder dislocation
    B. Due to abduction and external rotation
    C. More than 50% missed
    D. Hill Sach's lesion is seen
    E. Trough sign is due to fracture of posterior aspect of humeral head

34. **Sternum:**
    A. Manubrium ossifies in mid fetal life
    B. Mesosternum ossifies first
    C. The sternum ossifies from above downwards
    D. Ossification present at birth
    E. Segment 2 is ossifed before segment 4

35. **Anterior dislocation of shoulder:**
    A. Hill Sach's lesion is fracture of the inferior glenoid rim
    B. Bankart's lesion is fracture of the anterior aspect of humeral head
    C. Axillary artery is injured in anterior dislocation
    D. Light bulb sign is seen in anterior dislocation
    E. The humeral head rests under the coracoid process

36. **Scaphoid fracture complications:**
    A. Kienböck's disease
    B. Carpal instability
    C. Carpal tunnel syndrome
    D. Sudeck's dystrophy
    E. Madelung's deformity

37. **Scaphoid fractures:**
    A. Constitute 75% of carpal fractures
    B. X-rays are negative in 50% of cases
    C. The wrist is immobilised even in X-ray is negative
    D. In elderly patients, the fracture can take upto 12 weeks to be seen in plain X-rays
    E. The scaphoid has no periosteum

38. **Scaphoid fractures:**
    A. Ultrasound will show elevation of periosteum
    B. Disruption of cortex is the only ultrasound sign
    C. Four views are preformed in the standard scaphoid series
    D. If bone scan is negative and clinical suspicion is high, it should not be repeated within a week
    E. The fracture is unstable if the diastasis is more than 1 mm

39. **Sudeck's atrophy:**
    A. Soft tissue atrophied in early phases itself
    B. Disuse osteopenia has the same imaging appearance
    C. Ground glass appearance
    D. Subperiosteal bone absorption
    E. Sympathetic block treats the condition

40. **Scapula:**
    A. The coracoid process is a lateral projection of the scapular spine
    B. The acromion process is a lateral projection of the body of scapula
    C. The os acromiale is seen in 10% of normal population
    D. There are five secondary centers of ossification for scapula
    E. The scapula beings to ossify in eight weeks

41. **Scaphoid fractures:**
    A. All fractures are considered unstable
    B. The middle third is affected in 70% of cases
    C. The blood supply to scaphoid is from median artery and enters through proximal pole
    D. MRI is useful in assessing progress of treatment
    E. Foreshortening of scaphoid indicates DISI instability

42. **Bone marrow edema is seen normally in the following locations:**
    A. Posterior elements of vertebra
    B. Small bones of wrist
    C. Small bones of mid foot
    D. Epiphysis of long bones
    E. Diaphysis of long bones

43. **Causes of bone marrow edema:**
    A. Steroids
    B. Osteoid osteoma
    C. Synovitis
    D. Sympathetic dystrophy
    E. Transient osteoporosis of hip

44. **Bone marrow edema:**
    A. Bone bruise heals quicker since it occurs in the red marrow
    B. Bone bruise heals within 3 months
    C. Hyperemic bone bruises are more painful than other causes
    D. Bone edema may be seen in osteoarthritis
    E. Diffusion imaging is the best modality for assessing severity of bone edema

45. **Bone marrow edema:**
    A. High signal is seen in fat suppressed images
    B. Diffuse edema is seen in compression force
    C. In avulsion distraction injuries, the edema is seen parallel to the direction of stress
    D. Traction cysts result in sites of avulsion injury if weight bearing persists and trabecular non-union ensues
    E. Burst fractures result if persistent prolonged compression forces are applied

46. **Tibial plateau fractures:**
    A. Medial tibial condyle is commonly involved
    B. Valgus injury is more common than varus injury
    C. Lipohemarthrosis suggests communication of fracture with the articular surface
    D. Splitting occurs in younger patients
    E. Depression occurs in older patients

47. **Associated injuries of lateral tibial plateau fractures:**
    A. Posterior cruciate ligament
    B. Lateral collateral ligament
    C. Peroneal nerve
    D. Popliteal artery
    E. Lateral meniscus

48. **Burst fractures of spine:**
    A. Most common in the cervical spine
    B. The interpedicular distance is increased
    C. The posterior cortex of the vertebral body is not involved
    D. The spinal canal is not affected
    E. Caused by axial compression

49. **The following findings in a burst fracture indicate that it is unstable:**
    A. Neurologic signs
    B. Loss of 50% of vertebral body height
    C. Angulation of thoracolumbar junction more than 20 degrees
    D. Sagittal index more than 15 degrees
    E. Widened interpedicular distance

50. **Bone scan—Increased uptake is seen in:**
    A. Carcinoma of breast
    B. Calcium containing gallstones
    C. In kidney in the presence of right to left shunt
    D. Soft tissue in myositis ossificans
    E. Asbestos related pleural disease

51. **Indications for bone scan:**
    A. Shin splints
    B. Spondylolysis
    C. Plantar fasciitis
    D. Paget's disease
    E. Stress fracture

52. **Bone scan:**
    A. Within 2-6 hours after administration, there is uptake of 50% of isotope by skeletal system
    B. Optimal images are obtained 10 hours after administration
    C. The dose is 50 mCi
    D. Adsorption occurs to the organic phase of the bone
    E. New bone formation is the important factor deciding the isotope uptake

53. **Bone scan-normal activity:**
    A. Kidneys
    B. Facial bones in children
    C. Physes
    D. Bladder
    E. Soft tissue

54. **Bone scintigraphy:**
    A. Local extent of primary tumour can be demonstrated accurately
    B. Stress fracture can be demonstrated in the presence of a normal X-ray
    C. More than 70% of isotope is taken up by kidney
    D. In Paget's disease, osteoporosis circumscripta is cold
    E. In fracture femur, absence of uptake indicates lack of blood supply

55. **Positive bone scan in a 19-year-old male with severe pain in the leg may be due to:**
    A. Stress fracture
    B. Osteoid osteoma
    C. Arterial compression
    D. Chondromalacia patellae
    E. Brodie's abscess

56. **Increased uptake in bone scan may be seen in:**
    A. Normal breast
    B. Normal thymus
    C. Subphrenic abscess
    D. Acute myocardial infarct
    E. Myeloma

57. **Bone scan:**
    A. Blood pool images are obtained at 30 min after administration of isotope
    B. Increased uptake is seen with increased flow
    C. No renal excretion occurs with markedly increased uptake from any cause
    D. Sweat produces high uptake in axilla
    E. Tooth extraction causes high uptake

58. Bone scan with abnormal uptake in thorax:
A. Carcinoma of breast
B. Asbestos plaques
C. Alveolar microlithiasis
D. Chondrosarcoma
E. Pneumonia

59. Abnormal bone scan uptake in kidneys:
A. Renal vein thrombosis
B. Acute tubular necrosis
C. Pyelonephritis
D. Obstruction
E. Iron overload

60. Increased uptake of bone scan is seen in:
A. Rhabdomyolysis
B. Bismuth injection
C. Subdural haematoma
D. Hyperparathyroidism
E. Lymphedema

61. Bilateral symmetric increased uptake in the diaphysis:
A. Hypertrophic pulmonary osteoarthropathy
B. Fluorosis
C. Hypothyroidism
D. Shin splint
E. Engelmann's disease

62. Long segmental uptake in diaphysis:
A. Paget's
B. Osteogenesis imperfecta
C. Melorheostosis
D. Arterial injection
E. Fibrous dysplasia

63. Features of super scan:
A. Abnormal uptake in kidneys
B. Prominent uptake in the axial and appendicular skeleton
C. Visualisation of femoral cortices
D. Increased metaphyseal activity
E. Increased bone to soft tissue ratio

64. Causes of super scan:
A. Hyperthyroidism   B. Hypoparathyroidism
C. Osteoporosis   D. Osteomalacia
E. Renal osteodystrophy

65. **Increased uptake in bone scan is seen in:**
    A. Cerebral infarction
    B. Unstable angina pectoris
    C. Kidneys in gentamicin uptake
    D. Cirrhosis
    E. Accessory spleen

66. **Gallium scintigraphy increased bone activity seen in:**
    A. Sarcoma
    B. Lymphoma
    C. Septic arthritis
    D. Paget's disease
    E. Hyperparathyroidism

67. **Gallium useful in the following tumours:**
    A. Head and neck cancers
    B. GI tumours
    C. Hepatoma
    D. Melanoma
    E. Rhabdomyosarcoma

68. **Normal uptake in gallium seen in:**
    A. Thymus
    B. Kidneys
    C. Liver
    D. Breasts
    E. Spleen

ANSWERS

1. **A-F, B-T, C-T, D-T, E-F**

   The normal Bohler's angle is between 28 and 40 degrees. In fractures, the angle is reduced. Occasionally it may be reversed. Patellofemoral joint is the most common dislocation in the knee joint. Valgus stress with internal rotation causes lateral dislocation when there is medial blow to patella.

2. **A-F, B-F, C-T, D-T, E-T**

   Wedge compression is a feature of flexion injuries. Flexion and axial compression produces the tear drop fracture, which is a triangular fragment in the anteroinferior aspect of the vertebra. Neural arch and posterior column fractures are common in burst fractures which are due to axial compression. Locaked facets are seen due to flexion, rotation forces.

3. **A-T, B-T, C-F, D-T, E-T**

   Instability—Ruptured transverse ligament of atlas, Dens #, Burnt #, Bilateral facet dislocation, Hyperextension fracture dislocation, Hangman, extension tear drop, anterior subluxation, in children, subluxation upto 2 mm is normal, predontal space—< 3 mm in adult, < 5 mm in children, retropharyngeal space can be 22 mm in adults and 14 mm in children angulation more than 11 degrees in any space is abnormal, widening of spinous process space indicated posterior ligament our disruption.

4. **A-F, B-F, C-T, D-T, E-F**

   The mid third of clavicle is the most common segment to be fractured (65-80%). In fracture of the lateral third, the medial fragment is superior due to action of sternocleidomastoid and trapezius muscles. The lateral fragment is usually inferior due to the weight of shoulder upper limb. Injury to subclavian artery, subclavian vein, brachial plexus, pneumothorax are recognized complications of clavicular fractures.

5. **A-F, B-T, C-T, D-T, E-F**

   Sternoclavicular joint dislocation implies severe injury and is usually associated with fracture of ribs, injury to trachea, esophagus, SVC, brachiocephalic veins, phrenic nerve and vagus. Acromioclavicular dislocation, I—disruption of the acromioclavicular ligaments, with intact coracoclavicular ligaments, diagnosed only by stress view, with increased distance of acromioclavicular joint, II—disruption of acromioclavicular and conoid ligament, with increase in acromioclavicular distance in AP view, III— complete disruption of coracoclavicular and acromioclavicular ligaments, with increased coracoclavicular distance in AP film itself.

6. **A-T, B-F, C-F, D-T, E-T**
   Tear drop, Hangman's, Jefferson's, Bilateral locked facets, dens fracture and burst fractures are unstable. Type I is a fracture of tip.

7. **A-T, B-T, C-T, D-T, E-T**
   Fat pat sign in elbow refers to the displacement of the anterior and posterior fat pads in the elbow due to joint effusion. The most common cause is an intra-articular fracture. The other causes are:
   A. **Arthritis**—Hemophilia, RA,OA, neuropathic joint, gout, CPPD disease.
   B. **Infections**
   C. **Tumours**—Synovial sarcoma, osteoid osteoma, metastasis, leukaemia
   D. **Miscellaneous**—PVNS, synovial osteochondromatosis, osteochondritis dissecans

8. **A-F, B-F, C-T, D-T, E-T**
   Maisonneuve—medial malleolus fracture with proximal fibular shaft
   Jones—proximal 5th metatarsal shaft.

9. **A-T, B-T, C-T, D-F, E-F**
   Monteggia—fracture of proximal ulnar shaft with radial head dislocation.
   Galeazzi—fracture of distal radial shaft with distal radioulnar dislocation.
   Chance—commonly L2.

10. **A-F, B-T, C-F, D-F, E-T**
    Colle's—distal radius with dorsal displacement of fragment
    Smith's—ventral displacement of distal radius(reversed Colles)
    Barton's—fracture of dorsal lip of distal radius
    Hutchinson's fracture is also called Chauffeur's fracture.

11. **A-T, B-T, C-T, D-F, E-F**
    The blood supply to the talar dome enters through the distal talus and the talus is very prone for avascular necrosis.

12. **A-F, B-T, C-F, D-T, E-T**
    The head of the second and third metatarsals are the most common bones involved in stress fractures. In the early stages, there can be only subtle periosteal reaction to mark the stress fracture. Lisfranc's dislocation, can be homolateral or divergent. In homolateral, the dislocation is towards one direction. In divergent dislocation, they occur in opposite directions (first metatarsal shifted medially and rest of bones displaced laterally). Fracture of the base of the 2nd metatarsal is seen in both types.

13. **A-T, B-F, C-T, D-F, E-F**
Femoral shaft ossifies at 7 weeks of intrauterine life.The distal femoral epiphysis begins to ossify from nine months. The head-6 months, greater trochanter-4 years, lesser trochanter-puberty. These centers fuse with shaft at 18-20 years.

14. **A-F, B-F, C-F, D-F, E-F**
The normal alignment of foot—In AP view, the lateral border of the 1st MT is aligned with lateral border of medial cuneiform, the medial border of the 2nd MT is aligned with medial border of the intermediate cuneiform. In oblique view, the medial and lateral border of the third metatarsal are aligned with the medial and lateral border of the lateral cuneiform bone. The medial border of the 4th MT is aligned with the medial border of the cuboid bone. The lateral border of the 5th MT can project upto 5 mm beyond the lateral border of the cuboid bone. Mortise view of the ankle is performed in internal rotation. Talar dome avulsion is due to pull of tendons, since there are no muscles attached at this location.Avulsion of fifth metatarsal is due to pull of peroneus brevis tenson. Freiberg's infraction is seen in the head of the 2nd metatarsal bone.

15. **A-T, B-F, C-T, D-T, E-T**
Increased uptake in lungs after radiotherapy. Normal uptake is also seen in bowel and breast due to OC pills or antiemetics, liver, kidney, spleen.

16. **A-T, B-T, C-T, D-F, E-F**
Inability to weight bear, tenderness over tip and posterior aspect of medial and lateral malleolus are indications for X-ray of ankle in a setting of trauma.

17. **A-F, B-T, C-T, D-F, E-F**
Fractures of the lesser trochanter are less common than greater trochanter. Isolated fracture of the lesser trochanter and subtrochanteric region are likely to be pathological than primary. Scintigraphy can take upto three days for becoming positive, hence MRI is more sensitive from 2-3 hours. Impacted fractures produce less avascular necrosis.

18. **A-F, B-F, C-T, D-F, E-F**
Avascular necrosis is more common in subcapital fractures since the blood supply enters from the proximal part. Posterior dislocations are more common than anterior dislocations. CT scan, preferably with 3D reconstruction will be helpful for detecting the exact nature of the fracture of acetabular pillars. Mallet finger (baseball finger) is due to disruption of extensor tendon, involving

the distal interphalangeal joint. This is associated with flexion deformity and fracture fragment on the dorsal aspect of the phalanx. In volar plate avulsion, there is disruption of the volar plate and there is a fracture fragment on the volar aspect.

19. **A-F, B-T, C-F, D-F, E-T**
Stress fractures are of two types—Fatigue fractures—abnormal stress on a normal bone, Insufficiency fractures—Normal stress on abnormal bone, with low elastic resistance. MRI is as sensitive as bone scan and is more specific. Low signal is seen in the fractured area in both T1 and T2 images. This is surrounded by high signal area in both T1 and T2. Lower limb is more commonly affected. Shin splints are caused due to tearing of Sharpey's fibers which extend from the muscle, through periosteum into the bone.

20. **A-F, B-T, C-F, D-F, E-F**
The most common fracture fragment seen in the dorsal aspect of the wrist, is triquetral fracture which avulses at the site of attachment of the radiocarpal ligament. Scapholunate space normally measures 2 mm and is abnormal when more than 4 mm. Lunate dislocation is most common anteriorly. Foreshortening of the lunate is called Signet ring sign.

21. **A-T, B-F, C-T, D-F, E-T**
Inability to weight bear, tenderness over 5th metatarsal and navicular are indications.

22. **A-T, B-F, C-T, D-F, E-F**
Rolando's fracture is a comminuted fracture of the base of the 1st metacarpal. Boxer's fracture is a fracture of the base of 5th metacarpal, and can involve the base or distal shaft. Game-Keeper's or Skier's thumb is due to rupture of the ulnar collateral ligament. A routine AP film can show an avulsion fracture at the base of the proximal phalanx, but the injury is best seen when a radial stress view is preformed, when the MCP will show radial displacement due to torn ulnar collateral ligament. MRI used for sterneous lesion.

23. **A-T, B-T, C-T, D-T, E-F**
Isolated tenderness of patella, tender fibular head, over 55 years, inability to flex to 90 degrees and inability to weight bear are the indications.

24. **A-T, B-T, C-T, D-F, E-F**
Radial head dislocation in Monteggia, dislocation.

25. **A-T, B-F, C-T, D-T, E-F**
    Accidental injury, birth trauma, rickets, congenital incentivity to pain and paraplegia are other causes.

26. **A-T, B-F, C-F, D-F, E-T**
    Looser's zones are incomplete pseudofractures. Fracture line is not usually seen in stress fractures. Mild periosteal reaction and sclerosis are seen 1-2 weeks subsequent to onset of symptoms, but MRI and bone scan are more sensitive and are positive at the time of presentation. Transverse fracture in a long bone,called banana fracture is common in pathological fractures.

27. **A-F, B-T, C-T, D-T, E-T**
    Early mobilisation is essential in the management of Sudeck's atrophy. In 5% it is due to cervical disc disease. Associated with myocardial ischemia in 6%. All the joints in either hand or feet are affected.

28. **A-T, B-T, C-F, D-F, E-F**
    Trauma is the most common cause of Sudeck's and is seen in 0.01% of trauma.
    In majority, there is increased uptake in the flow, blood pool and delayed images. In 20% there may decreased uptake in all phases. Osteopenia can develop in two or three weeks.

29. **A-F, B-F, C-F, D-F, E-T**
    Anterior superior iliac spine—Sartorius and tensor, Inferior iliac spine—rectus femoris.
    Greater trochanter—gluteal muscles, Lesser trochanter—psoas muscle
    Ischial tuberosity—hamstrings

30. **A-F, B-T, C-F, D-F**
    Mandibular metastases are uncommon, due to paucity of red marrow.

31. **A-F, B-T, C-T, D-F, E-T**
    There are five types
    I—minimal displacement, no anterior displacement, no soft tissue
    II—greater displacement, anterior displacement, no disc narrowing
    III—same as above, with disc narrowing
    IV—fracture on one side and perched facet on other side
    V—communuted vertebra

32. **A-T, B-F, C-T, D-T, E-F**
    Type IV is unstable, because of bilateral disruption of lateral column. In AP, interfacetal joint spaces are seen. Spinous process

is in midline. In lateral view, double outline is seen due to lack of superimposition of posterior margin of articular masses at same level. Anterior listhesis and disk space narrowing can be seen. Rotation of vertebra at affected levels and above it are seen.

33. **A-F, B-F, C-T, D-F, E-F**
Anterior dislocation more than 95% of shoulder dislocations.
It is due to internal rotation and is common in direct trauma or seizures.
Fracture is seen in the anterior aspect of humeral head when it hits the posterior glenoid rim.

34. **A-T, B-F, C-T, D-T, E-F**
The manubrium ossifies first, at 6 months, followed by meso-sternum. The mesosternum ossfies from above downwards with segment 2 ossifying before segment 4. The ossification is present at birth.

35. **A-F, B-F, C-T, D-F, E-T**
In anterior dislocation the humeral head is in abduction and external rotation. The Hill Sach's lesion is fracture of the postero-lateral aspect of humeral head due to impact with anterior glenoid margin and Bankart's lesion is fracture of the inferior glenoid rim. Light bulb sign is seen in posterior dislocation due to internal rotation of humeral head.

36. **A-F, B-T, C-T, D-T, E-F**

37. **A-T, B-F, C-T, D-T, E-T**
Scaphoid fracture is the most common carpal fracture. X-ray can be negative in upto 25% of cases. X-rays can take upto 7-14 days to become positive and in elderly can take 2-12 weeks. Malunion, nonunion, avascular necrosis, arthritis are other complications.

38. **A-F, B-T, C-T, D-F, E-T**
Because of absence of periosteum, subperiosteal haematoma and lifting of periosteum which are commonly seen in other fractures is not seen. The standard views are AP, lateral, oblique and ulnar deviation.

39. **A-F, B-T, C-T, D-T, E-T**
Soft tissue swelling is seen in the early phases. But atrophy is seen in chronic stage after six months. Disuse osteopenia is difficult to differentiate. Ground glass appearance is due to resorption of one at endosteal, subperiosteal, intracortical, subchondral levels.

40. **A-F, B-F, C-T, D-F, E-T**

The coracoid is lateral projection of body and acromion, of spine of scapula.

There are two centers for glenoid fossa, two for medial border and one for inferior pole of scapula.These appear at puberty and fuse by 25 years. The center for coracoid appears at first year and fuses at 14 years. Os acromiale is a persistent ossification center at end of acromian. It is associated with shoulder impingement and rotator cliff tear.

41. **A-T, B-T, C-F, D-T, E-T**

Although fracture separation less than 1mm is considered stable, all fractures should be treated potentially unstable and treated accordingly. The waist is affected in 70%, the proximal pole in 20% and distal pole in 10%. Blood supply enters through distal pole through radial artery.

42. **A-F, B-T, C-T, D-F, E-F**

Bone marrow edema is commonly due to increased capillary leakage and hence seen in cancellous bones with rich capillary supply, such as metaphysis of long bones, vertebral body (not the posterior elements, small bones of the wrist and mid foot).

43. **A-T, B-T, C-T, D-T, E-T**

Causes of bone marrow edema

Hyperemic—increased blood flow—osteomyelitis and synovitis

Congestive—decreased vascular drainage—Increased intra-medullary pressure (steroid induced avascular necrosis, transient osteoporosis of hip), capillary thrombosis

Traumatic—most common cause

Tumours—osteoid osteoma(inflammatory mediators), aggressive tumours.

44. **A-T, B-T, C-F, D-T, E-T**

Bone edema in traumatic setting is called bone bruise. The trauma may be acute of repetitive chronic trauma, such as osteoarthritis. Only when associated with cortical bone destruction, it will be labelled as fracture. Hyperemic bone bruises are less painful than other causes, such as tumour or trauma which cause destruction of neurovascular structures. Diffusion imaging confirms increased diffusion co efficient and is the most sensitive indicator of severe marrow injury.

45. **A-T, B-T, C-F, D-T, E-T**

T1—hypo, T2—hyper, STIR and Fat suppression-hyper, DW—increased Diff co-efficient, Gd—delayed enhancement. **Impaction** forces cause concertina like globular edema in contrecoup surfaces, and compression fracture if severe. **Distraction** causes edema perpendicular to the direction of stress and avulsion fractures if severe. **Shear** causes oblique areas of edema and will result in oblique fractures if severe.

46. **A-F, B-T, C-T, D-T, E-T**
    Lateral tibial plateau is commonly injured than the medial plateau, as the valgus injuries are common, since the other leg protects medially. Injury is commonly due to axial loading and common in middle aged and old patients. Splitting occurs more in younger patients and depression occurs more in older patients.

47. **A-F, B-F, C-T, D-F, E-T**
    Anterior cruciate ligament, medial collateral ligament, peroneal nerve, lateral meniscus are commonly injured in lateral tibial plateau injuries. Posterior cruciate ligament, lateral collateral ligament, popliteal artery and medial meniscus are involved in medial tibial plateau injuries.

48. **A-F, B-T, C-F, D-F, E-T**
    Burst fracture of spine is caused by axial compression. This is a comminuted fracture with involvement of the posterior aspect of the vertebral body and fracture fragments are often found in the spinal canal, which is confirmed by CT scans. Most common location is the dorsolumbar junction. The interpedicular distance is increased and is best assessed in AP views.

49. **A-T, B-T, C-T, D-T, E-F**
    Neurological signs are due to involvement of posterior elements with involvement of the spinal canal or entrapment of the nerves within the fracture fragments. Sagittal index is measured by subtracting baseline sagittal curve from the lateral Cobb angle. Lateral Cobb angle is obtained in lateral films by joining a line exending from the inferior end plate of the involved vertebra and the inferior end plate of the vertebra superior to the involved vertebra. The normal value is 5 degrees for thoracic spine, 0 degree for dorsolumbar vertebrae and 10 degrees for lumbar vertebra.

50. **A-T, B-F, C-T, D-T, E-T**
    Myocardial infarction, cerebral infarction, malignant plenal effusion, inflammatory breast cancer, liver metastasis, liver necrosis are other cancer.

51. **A-T, B-T, C-T, D-T, E-T**
    The extent of Paget's disease can be assessed using bone scan. Osteomyelitis and avascular necrosis are other conditions that can be diagnosed by bone scans, earlier than radiographs.

52. **A-T, B-F, C-F, D-T, E-T**
   99 m technetium labeled methylene diphosphonate is the isotope used in bone scan. 20-25 mCi is the dose administered. Within 2-6 hours, 50% of this isotope is taken up by the bone. Adsorption to the mineral phase of the bony matrix is thought to be the mechanism. The uptake depends on the blood supply to the bone and more important, new bone formation. Optimal images with better target to background ratio, is obtained 2-6 hours after administration. Image quality may be further improved by intake a large amount of fluid.

53. **A-T, B-T, C-T, D-T, E-T**
   Uptake in bladder, kidneys and soft tissue are normal. In children high uptake is seen in the active growth plates and flat facial bones. Inferior angle of scapula, cartilages, ripples, renal pelvis, bladder diverticulum are also normal.

54. **A-F, B-T, C-F, D-F, E-T**
   MRI is more sensitive than bone scan or assessing the extent of tumour. Stress fractures are seen very late in plain X-rays. Bone scans are very sensitive. In Paget's, osteoporosis circumscripta is the active lytic stage in skull and hence is very hot. In fracture femur, normal bone scan uptake indicates normal vascularity. Absence of uptake indicates loss of blood supply either due to increased intracapsular pressure, and this normalizes in 3 to 5 months. Persistence cold spot indicates development of avascular necrosis.

55. **A-T, B-T, C-F, D-F, E-T**
   Shint splints, osteomyelitis, osteosarcoma, Ewing's are other causes.

56. **A-T, B-F, C-T, D-T, E-F**
   Myeloma usually has no uptake.

57. **A-T, B-T, C-F, D-T, E-T**

58. **A-T, B-T, C-T, D-T, E-F**
   Breast cancer, malignant pleural efussion.

59. **A-T, B-T, C-T, D-T, E-T**

60. **A-T, B-F, C-T, D-T, E-T**
   Seen in iron dextran and meperidine injections.

61. **A-T, B-F, C-F, D-T, E-T**

62. **A-T, B-T, C-T, D-T, E-T**
   Also in venous stasis, Vitamin A toxicity and osteomyelitis

63. **A-F, B-F, C-T, D-T, E-T**
    No uptake in kidneys. Prominent uptake in axial skeleton, especially in skull, mandible, costochondral junctions and sternum. Increased periarticular activity is also seen.

64. **A-T, B-F, C-F, D-T, E-T**
    Paget's disease, myelosclerosis, myelofibrosis, leukemia, mastocytosis, metastasis, waldenstorms are other causes.

65. **A-T, B-T, C-T, D-F, E-F**

66. **A-T, B-F, C-T, D-T, E-F**
    Also in active osteomyelitis, cellulitis and rheumatoid arthritis.

67. **A-F, B-F, C-T, D-T, E-T**
    Also useful in non-small cell cancers, Burkitt's lymphoma.Gallium is not useful in head and neck tumours, GI tumours, gynaecological tumours, pediatric tumours and breast cancer.

68. **A-T, B-T, C-T, D-T, E-T**
    Breasts—lactation, pregnancy, menarche, estrogens
    Thymus—in children
    Spleen—in splenomegaly

6 Shoulder, Elbow and Wrist

1. **Shoulder:**
   A. The clavicle does not have a medullary cavity
   B. The clavicle is the first bone to ossify in humans
   C. The rhomboid fossa is seen in 15% of population in the inferomedial aspect of the clavicles
   D. The coracoclavicular ligament has two components
   E. Supraclavicular nerves can pass through the mid portion of clavicle

2. **Acromioclavicular joint:**
   A. A distance of 3 mm between the inferior margin of acromion and superior surface of humerus is indicative of supraspinatus tear
   B. A fibrocartilagenous disc is seen in the joint
   C. The principal stablising influence on the joint are the coraclavicular ligaments
   D. Inferior subluxation of clavicle is produced in conoid and trapezoid ligament disruption
   E. Acromioclavicular ligament is a strong capsule around the joint

3. **Anatomy:**
   A. All the lymphatic from the hand drain into the lateral pectoral group of lymph nodes
   B. The axillary vein lies lateral to the neurovascular bundle in the axilla
   C. There are five groups of axillary lymph nodes
   D. The anatomical neck of humerus is situated below the surgical neck
   E. The profunda brachii artery runs through the radial groove

4. **Shoulder joint:**
   A. The joint capsule is lax inferiorly
   B. The long head of biceps runs under the intertubercular ligament

C. The transverse ligament of humerus is an extension of the coracohumeral ligament
D. The subscapular bursa separates the scapular neck and subscapularis
E. Subscapularis bursa is formed by herniation of shoulder joint synovial membrane through a defect in glenohumeral ligament

5. **Shoulder joint arthrography can assess the following:**
   A. Joint volume
   B. Bony configuration of humeral head and· glenoid
   C. Axillary recess
   D. Tendon sheath of biceps short head
   E. Subscapularis tendon

6. **Muscles** and their insertion:
   A. Supraspinatus—middle facet of greater tubercle of humerus
   B. Subscapularis—inferior facet of greater tubercle of humerus
   C. Infraspinatus—inferior facet of greater tubercle of humerus
   D. Teres minor—middle facet of greater tubercle of humerus
   E. Shoulder joint is composed of three joints

7. **Rotator cuff pathology:**
   A. In ultrasound of shoulder, for visualizing the supraspinatus tendon, the shoulder is placed in adduction and internal rotation
   B. MRI is better than ultrasound for diagnosis of small tears
   C. Subtle areas of calcification are seen better in ultrasound than MRI
   D. High resolution ultrasound can be used to detect pathology in bone
   E. Ultrasound should be avoided directly over the site of clinical pain

8. **Features of shoulder arthrogram suggesting rotator cuff tear:**
   A. Filling of subacromial bursa
   B. Filling of subscapular busa
   C. Increased volume of joint cavity
   D. Irregularity of the outer border of the clavicle
   E. Filling of the bicipital bursa

9. **MRI of shoulder:**
   A. Is performed ideally in prone position
   B. In supine position, the arm is placed over the abdomen
   C. High signal in the tissues may be caused due to coil burnout
   D. The coronal oblique image is oriented along the supraspinatus tendon and muscle
   E. Transverse images are ideal for demonstrating labral capsular complex

10. **MRI of shoulder:**
    A. Field of view of 14 cm or less is required
    B. T1W images are optimal for visualising the joint anatomy
    C. The coronal plane is perpendicular to the glenoid plane
    D. Oblique coronal images are acquired parallel to the supraspinatus muscle as visualised in axial images
    E. Off center FOV is essential

11. **Shoulder joint views:**
    A. Strip view is performed in the seated position
    B. The tube is tilted cephalad in strip view
    C. The trans scapular view is centered on the head of the humerus and long axis of scapula
    D. Striker's view is used for visualizing Hill Sach's lesion
    E. The humerus is tilted 45 degrees from horizontal in Striker's views

12. **MRI of shoulder—Technical features:**
    A. Motion artefacts are common in the high field magnets
    B. Mid field scanners are adequate for a standard shoulder examination
    C. 3D images have limited soft tissue contrast resolution
    D. Echoplanar images allow fast 3D acquisition and good contrast
    E. If FSE is used, both non fat suppressed and fat suppressed sequences should be obtained

13. **In shoulder MRI, contrast enhancment is useful in following situations:**
    A. Partial articular surface tears
    B. Differentiating tendonitis and tears
    C. Postoperative shoulder
    D. Capsular anatomy
    E. Labral anatomy

14. **MRI of shoulder:**
    A. Sagittal oblique images are ideal for evaluation of coracoacromial arch
    B. Transverse images are ideal for labral capsular complex
    C. Acromioclavicular joint are best assessed in axial plane
    D. Superior and inferior portions of glenoid labrum are best assessed in coronal oblique plane
    E. Subscapularis tendon is best assessed in the axial plane

15. **Rotator cuff disease:**
    A. Type 1 acromion is flat
    B. Type 2 acromion is hooked
    C. Type 3 acromion is associated with 80% of rotator cuff tears
    D. Type 2 acromion is rarely associated with tear
    E. Acromial shape is best appreciated in the coronal oblique images

16. **Rotator cuff tear:**
    A. Subacromial osteophytes are a predisposing factor for impingement syndrome
    B. Deltoid tendon insertion in the inferior aspect of acromion can mimic a subacromial spur
    C. High signal in the supraspinatus tendon is always indicative of tear
    D. Magic angle effect produces high signal mimicking tear
    E. External rotation of shoulder produces an artifactual high signal in supraspinatus

17. **Rotator cuff tear:**
    A. Differentiating partial tear and tendinopathy is imperative for management
    B. Presence of a visible separation in the supraspinatus, is the only absolute criterion in the diagnosis of complete tear
    C. Fluid in the glenohumeral joint and subacromial space suggests complete tear
    D. Fluid in subacromial space suggests complete tear
    E. Decrease of subdeltoid fat plane may be useful for diagnosing tear or tendinopathy

18. **MRI of shoulder joint:**
    A. Labral tear is frequently associated with glenoid cyst
    B. The labrum is a triangular structure
    C. Tear may be mimicked by plane between labrum and glenohumeral ligaments
    D. SLAP lesions are best seen in axial images
    E. Bankart's lesion is best seen with capsular distension

19. **Glenohumeral instability is caused by:**
    A. Bankart's lesion
    B. Hill Sach's lesion
    C. Labral tear
    D. Capsular avulsion
    E. Glenohumeral ligamental avulsion

20. **MRI of shoulder:**
    A. MRI can differentiate partial from complete tear
    B. Axial plane is best to demonstrate subscapularis tear
    C. Tears commonly happen just proximal to musculotendinous junction
    D. Contrast arthrography is better seen for adhesive capsulitis
    E. Infraspinatus is the most common tendon to be torn in rotator cuff injury

21. **The rotator cuff tear:**
    A. The most common site is at the tendon muscle junction
    B. Teres minor tear is best imaged in coronal section
    C. Adhesive capsulitis is better seen in conventional arthrography rather than MR
    D. CT requires contrast to show the labrum
    E. It is easy to distinguish partial tear from tendonitis

22. **Triangular fibrocartilage complex comprises of:**
    A. Ulnar collateral ligament
    B. Dorsal radioulnar ligament
    C. Extensor carpi ulnaris sheath
    D. Volar radioulnar ligament
    E. Meniscus

23. **Bones of upper limb:**
    A. In 10% of people, a supratrochlear foramen is present
    B. The supracondylar spur is seen 10 cm proximal to the medial epicondyle
    C. The supracondylar spur is seen in about 3% of individuals
    D. Median nerve palsy is a recognized complication of supracondylar spur
    E. Morphologically, the supracondylar spur is a remnant of the inferior portion of brachialis

24. **Bones of upper limb:**
    A. The common extensor origin is in medial epicondyle
    B. The center for head of humerus appears at 3 years
    C. The centers of ossification of upper end of humerus fuse with the shaft in 6 years
    D. The radial ossification center appears in 1 year
    E. The ulnar ossification center fuseds at 20 years

25. **Ossification of elbow:**
    A. The capitellum is formed at 3 years
    B. The radial head and medial epicondyle are formed in 5 years
    C. Trochlea is not formed in 10 years
    D. Medial epicondyle is the third ossification center to form
    E. The centers fuse at 13 years

26. **Insertion of elbow muscles:**
    A. Triceps—olecranon
    B. Biceps—deep fascia of forearm
    C. Brachialis—coronoid process
    D. Biceps—radial tuberosity
    E. Coracobrachialis—radial head

27. **Elbow:**
    A. The bicipital aponeurosis is deep to the median cubital vein and brachial artery
    B. The fibers of annular ligament are attached to ulna
    C. The ulnar collateral ligament is seen as a single structure in MRI
    D. The radial collateral ligament is a thickening of the elbow joint capsule
    E. The elbow joint capsule is attached to the middle aspect of olecranon

28. **Upper limb bones:**
    A. The carrying angle is higher in females
    B. The males have carrying angle of 168 degrees
    C. If a line is drawn through the anterior end of humerus, it should intersect the posterior 1/3rd of the humeral capitellum
    D. Anterior fat pad is normal in 15% of normal population
    E. The interosseus membrane of forearm arises from the median groove of radius and is well seen in MRI

29. **Upper limb:**
    A. There are 15 muscles in the extensor compartment of the forearm
    B. Normally, The inferior radioulnar joint communicates with the carpal joint
    C. The radius articulates with lunate, scaphoid and triquetral bones
    D. The triquetrum is indirect contact with ulna
    E. The radiocarpal and mid carpal joint communicate in 50% of individuals

30. **Contents of the main compartment of carpal tunnel:**
    A. Flexor carpi radialis
    B. Flexor digitorum superficialis
    C. Flexor digitorum profundus
    D. Ulnar artery
    E. Flexor pollicis longus

31. **The flexor retinaculum is attached to the following structures:**
    A. The hook of the hamate
    B. Scaphoid tubercle
    C. Trapezium ridge
    D. Pisiform
    E. Ulnar styloid

32. **Ossification of carpal bones:**
    A. Pisiform is the last bone to form
    B. Capitate 1 year
    C. Triquetrum 3 years
    D. Trapezoid 4 years
    E. Pisiform 10 years

33. **Hand:**
    A. The primary movement of thumb takes place in the carpometacarpal joint
    B. The most common sesamoid bone in hand is in the tendon of flexor pollicis longus
    C. The most common sesamoid bone in the wrist is the os radiale
    ⁎ externum
    D. Bone age is estimated using X-rays of right hand
    E. There are six extensor compartments of tendons

34. **Types of joints:**
    A. Metacarpal joints—hinged synovial
    B. Shoulder—ball and socket
    C. Elbow—ball and socket
    D. Inferior radioulnar joint—pivot synovial
    E. Acromioclavicular joint—fibrous

35. **The compartments of the extensor compartment of the wrist:**
    A. There are seven compartments
    B. The first compartment is on the radial side
    C. The third and fourth compartments are separated by the extensor tubercle of radius
    D. The extensor pollicis longus tenson is seen in the first compartment
    E. Extensor digiti minimi is seen in the sixth compartment

36. **De Quervains tenosynovitis:**
    A. More common in females
    B. Bilateral in 70%
    C. Affects the sixth compartment of wrists
    D. Caused due to trauma during radial deviation of wrist
    E. Pain is present over ulnar styloid

37. **Common causes of carpal tunnel syndrome:**
    A. Pregnancy
    B. Menopause
    C. Hypertrophy of muscles
    D. Accessory abductor digiti minimi
    E. Accessory flexor digitorum superficialis

38. **MRI features of carpal tunnel syndrome:**
    A. Flattening of median nerve
    B. Volar bowing of flexor retinaculum
    C. Enlarged median nerve inside the tunnel
    D. Tiny pockets of fluid collection along the median nerve
    E. Low signal within the median nerve in T2W imags

39. **Carpal tunnel syndrome:**
    A. Nerve conduction studies are 90% sensitive
    B. High signal intensity in median neve is specific for carpal tunnel syndrome
    C. Persistent median artery is a recognised cause of capal tunnel syndrome
    D. The most common peripheral nerve entrapment syndrome
    E. Atrophy is seen in the hypothenar eminence

40. **Carpal tunnel syndrome:**
    A. MRI is more useful in postoperative then preoperative
    B. 2% have persistent symptoms after surgery
    C. Incomplete division of retinaculum is a common cause
    D. Nocturnal paraesthesias are seen
    E. The nerve enhances in contrast scans

41. **Ganglions:**
    A. The most common hand tumour
    B. Formed due to remodelling of fibrous joint capsule
    C. Most common in females
    D. Contain mucin
    E. Enhance with contrast

42. **Ganglion:**
    A. Multiloculated
    B. 70% seen in the dorsal aspect of wrist
    C. Intraosseous ganglions show low signal in T1 and T2 images
    D. Ganglions are in the diaphysis of bones
    E. Intraosseous ganglion show a sclerotic rim

43. **Kienböck's disease:**
    A. Males commonly affected
    B. Seen in older women more than 60 years old
    C. Carpal tunnel syndrome is a clinical presentation
    D. Not seen in those with positive ulnar variance
    E. X-rays are normal in Stage I disease

44. Kienböck's disease:
  A. Compression fractures seen in stage I disease
  B. Synovitis is seen in early stages
  C. Associated with Madelung's deformity
  D. In stage IIIB, entire long axis of scaphoid not seen in coronal view
  E. Osteoarthritis is seen in stage IV

45. Recognised causes of olecranon bursitis:
  A. Synovial osteochondromatosis
  B. Rheumatoid arthritis
  C. Steroid
  D. Dialysis
  E. Osteoarthritis

46. Miner's elbow:
  A. Olecranon bursa is seen at birth normally
  B. Second most common bursitis in the body after the infra-patellar bursa
  C. Associated with triceps tendon rupture
  D. Associated with Staphylococcus aureus infection
  E. In rheumatoid arthritis, communicates with the elbow joint

ANSWERS

1. **A-T, B-T, C-F, D-T, E-T**
The clavicle ossifies in the first month of fetal life. Secondary centers appear at 16 years at the medial end, fuse at 25 years. The rhomboid fossa is seen in 5% and it represents the origin of the rhomboid ligament, which extends to the first costal cartilage. Coracoclavicular ligament has the conoid ligament medially and trapezoid ligament laterally, which extend from inferolateral surface of clavicle to coracoid process.

2. **A-T, B-T, C-T, D-F, E-F**
Distance less than 5 mm indicates supraspinatus tear. Conoid and trapezoid ligament disruption produces superior subluxation. Acromioclavicular ligament produces a poorly formed capsule.

3. **A-F, B-F, C-T, D-F, E-T**
The lymphatics drain into lateral pectoral group, except from the first webspace and thumb which drain into the infraclavicular group. The axillary vein lies medial to the neurovascular bundle. Lateral, subscapular, pectoral, central and apical are the five lymph nodal groups. The surgical neck lies below the anatomical neck of humerus. The radial nerve and produnda brachii artery run through the radial groove.

4. **A-T, B-T, C-T, D-T, E-T**
The coracohumeral ligament runs from undersurface of coracoid to lesser tubercle of humerus and then continues as the intertubercular or the transverse ligament.

5. **A-T, B-T, C-T, D-F, E-T**
Long head of biceps, supraspinatus tendon and subscapularis bursa are other assessed structures.

6. **A-F, B-F, C-F, D-F, E-T**
Supraspinatus, infrapinatus and teres minor insert into the superior, middle and inferior facets of the greater tubercle of humerus. Subscapularis inserts into the lesser tubercle of humerus. The shoulder has three joints, the glenohumeral, acromioclavicular and scapulothoracic joints. The sternoclavicular joint is also associated with the shoulder. Teres major—medial lip of bicipital groove.

7. **A-T, B-F, C-T, D-F, E-F**
MRI and ultrasound are useful in evaluation of rotator cuff pathologies. Ultrasound of the supraspinatus tendon is done with the shoulder in internal rotation and adduction. Ultrasound has been proved to be more sensitive than MRI in diagnosis of small

tears and shows good correlation with surgical findings. Subtle areas of calcification are better seen than MRI, comparable to plain X-ray. Ultrasound has the advantage of being able to scan exactly over the site of clinical pain and tenderness and scanning the contralateral limb. Although fractures, osteophytes and erosions can be seen sometimes in ultrasound, it is not reliable to diagnose bony lesions.

8. **A-T, B-F, C-F, D-F, E-F**
   Full thickness tear is seen at contrast entering through the defect in the cuff into subacromial subdeltoid bursa. Partial thickness tears, extension of contrast into tendon, MR arthrography has replaced conventional arthrogram.

9. **A-T, B-F, C-T, D-T, E-T**
   MRI of shoulder is done ideally in the prone oblique position, which minimizes motion artefacts. If done in the supine position, the arm is placed by the side in an external rotation position and not over the abdomen to avoid breathing artefacts. Images are acquired in coronal oblique (along the line of supraspinatus muscle and tendon), sagittal(perpendicular to supraspinatus and parallel to glenoid and transverse planes. T1, T2, STIR coronal, T2 FLASH axial and T1 sagittal images are acquired. The common artifacts are breathing and coil burn out. Coil burn out results in high signal emanating in superficial tissues and progressively decreasing deeper.

10. **A-T, B-F, C-T, D-T, E-T**
    Because of the lateral location of the shoulder joint, the field of view is positioned off center and a FOV of 14 cm or less is required to get high resolution. T1W images alone are not optimal for demonstrating the joint anatomy as most of the structures are small. T2, STIR are other useful sequences. The coronal plane of shoulder is perpendicular to the face of the glenoid fossa and sagittal plane is parallel to it. The oblique coronal images are acquired parallel to the supraspinatus muscle and tendon and this is identified with the help of the axial images.

11. **A-T, B-T, C-T, D-T, E-F**
    Strip view—Axial view in those with limited shoulder abduction-patient is seated and holds film above shoulder. Lean's back by 15 degrees. Tube in ground and cephalad.
    Striker's view—for posterior aspect of head and cortical lesions-patient is supine and humerus is 90 degrees. Centered on humeral head, angled 25 degrees cephalad.

Trans-scapular view—centered on head of humerus and long axis of scapula. The arcs formed by glenoid, humeral head and acromioclavicular joint with acromion are seen.

12. **A-T, B-T, C-T, D-T, E-T**

High field units give high signal to noise ratios, high spatial resolution and decreased scan time but have more motion artefacts. Mid field scanners can give as good performance as high field units, if it has good coil design, high field uniformity and eddy current compensation. 3D images provide useful information, but acquisition in gradient echo mode to reduce time, results in poor soft tissue contrast. This is compensated by using newer gradient echo sequences or echoplanar sequences which give good soft tissue contrast. If FSE is used, a non fat suppressed sequence (distinguishes tear and severe degeneration) and fat suppressed sequence (for fluid, edema and bone changes) should be obtained.

13. **A-T, B-T, C-T, D-T, E-T**

Contrast MRI is better in postoperative shoulder, since gradient echo images will produce significant magnetic susceptibility artefacts.

14. **A-T, B-T, C-F, D-T, E-T**

Coronal oblique images are good for assessing supraspinatus tendon, subacromial region, acromioclavicular region and superior and inferior portion of glenoid. The sagittal oblique images are used for evaluating the coracoacromial arch and subacromio-clavicular issues. Axial images are used for evaluating the labral capsular complex which includes the glenoid labrum, joint capsule, glenohumeral ligaments and subscapularis tendon.

15. **A-T, B-F, C-T, D-F, E-F**

Acromial shape is best seen in the sagittal oblique images. There are three types of acromion, Type 1 is a flat acromion. Type 2 has a concave inferior surface and Type 3 is hooked, with an anterior hook in the anterior border of a curved acromion. Type 1 is not associated with any tear. 80% of tears are seen in association with type 3 acromion and 20% with type 2.

16. **A-T, B-T, C-F, D-T, E-F**

Osteoarthritis of the acromioclavicular joint, with subacromial osteophytes narrow the subacromial space, and causes impingement. The deltoid tenson insertion on the inferior aspect of the acromion, if not imaged in continuity, may mimic a subacromial spur. High singal wihin supraspinatus tendon is suggestive of rotator cuff disease. High signal may also be seen in T1 weighted images due to magic angle effect, partial volume averaging and internal rotation causing overlap of tendons and long head of biceps tendon as it passes through the rotator cuff. These artefactual high signal in T1 do not show high signal in T2 weighted images.

17. **A-F, B-T, C-T, D-F, E-T**
Visible disruption of the supraspinatus tendon, with or without retraction is the absolute sign of complete tear of supraspinatus tendon. Fluid seen concomitantly in subacromial space and glenohumeral space is another sign. Isolated fluid in subacromial space without a defect in supraspinatus tendon is suggestive, but not pathognomonic as bursitis or steroid injection can give a similar finding. High signal or partial disruption of tendon suggests either a partial tear of tendinopathy, both of which cannot be reliably distinguished by MRI, which anyway is not imperative as both are managed conservatively.

18. **A-F, B-F, C-T, D-F, E-T**
The labrum is best seen in axial images and can be triangular or cresenteric or round or absent. Tear may be mimicked by undercutting of the base of the labrum by the glenoid articular cartilage and the cleavage plane between middle and inferior glenohumeral ligaments and the labrum. The tear may be associated with glenoid cyst, but not very frequently. SLAP (Superior labrum, anterior, posterior), tears are seen in athletes performing overhead actions and are seen best in coronal oblique images. The clinical significance of these lesions is not known. Bankart's lesion, which is capsular stripping with bony changes is seen best with capsular distension. So it is better seen if there is a joint effusion or in MR arthrography.

19. **A-T, B-T, C-T, D-T, E-T**
Congenital—glenoid dysplasia, Ehlers-Danlos syndrome
Trauma—bone, rotator cuff, labrum, capsule, ligaments' labral tears
Neuromuscular—stroke, brachial plexus injuries, encephalitis
Multidirectional instability—loose capsule/ligaments/labrum
Anterior—Labral/IGHL injury, posterior—Hill Sach's.

20. **A-T, B-T, C-F, D-T, E-F**
Tear is common at the critical zone due to junction of two vascular zones. Some studies show a predilection close to insertion site.

21. **A-T, B-F, C-T, D-T, E-F**
Teres minor and subscapularis tears are best seen in axial images. Partial thickness tear and tendonitis show high signal within the tendon and ponce cannot be differentiated easily.

22. **A-T, B-T, C-T, D-T, E-T**
    The triangular fibrocartilage complex consists of triangular fibrocartilage, ulnar carpal meniscus, dorsal and volar radioulnar ligament, ulnar colateral ligament and sheath of extensor carpi ulnaris tendon.

23. **A-T, B-F, C-F, D-T, E-F**
    Supracondylar spur is seen in less than 1% of population. It is the remnant of the inferior portion of coracobrachialis. Seen 5 cm proximal to medial epicondyle, sometimes a ligament of Struther's connects the spur to the medial epicondyle. Median artery and brachial artery may run under this ligament, which may compress on these structures.

24. **A-T, B-F, C-F, D-T, E-F**
    The secondary centers for head, greater tubercle and lesser tubercle are formed in 1, 3, 5 years. They fuse together in 6 years and fuse with shaft at 20 years. The radial secondary center appears at 1 year, fuses at 20 years. Ulna secondary center appears at 5 years and fuses at 17 years.

25. **A-F, B-T, C-T, D-T, E-F**
    CRITOL is the mnemonic.
    Capitellum—1 year,
    Radial head—5 years,
    Internal epicondyle—5 years,
    Trochlea—11 years,
    Olecranon—12 years,
    Lateral epicondyle—13 years
    These fuse at 15-17 years.

26. **A-T, B-T, C-T, D-T**
    Biceps divides into two and inserts into the deep fascia of forearm and the radial tuberosity. Coracobrachialis—middle 1/3rd, medial aspect of humerus.

27. **A-F, B-T, C-T, D-T, E-F**
    The bicipital aponeurosis separates the median cubital vein and brachial artery. The joint capsule is attached above the olecranon, radial and cornoid fossa above and below to the olecranon and coronoid processes.The radial collateral ligament is a lateral thickening of the joint capsule and blends with the annular ligament. The annular ligament surrounds the head of radius and is attached to the ulna and blends with the radial collateral ligament laterally.

28. **A-T, B-T, C-F, D-T, E-T**
    Carrying angle is 168 in males and 170 in females. The anterior humeral cortical line, should pass only through the anterior 1/3rd of capitellum.

29. **A-F, B-F, C-T, D-F, E-T**
    There are 12 muscles in the extensor compartment. The radioulnar joint normally does not communicate with the radiocarpal joint, unless there is rupture of the triangular fibrocartilage.Although it was initially believed that there is no communication between radioulnar, radiocarpal and mid-carpal joints, recent studies demonstrate presence of communication between Radioulnar and radiocarpal in 30%, between radiocarpal and mid-carpal in 50% and between radioulnar and pisiform bursa in 50%. The radius articulates with scaphoid and lunate and with triquetrum in ulnar deviation.
    The ulnar is separated from carpal bones by the articular disc.

30. **A-F, B-T, C-T, D-F, E-T**
    Flexor carpi radialis lies in a separate compartment, separate from the other structures in the carpal tunnel. Ulnar artery lies superficial to the flexor retinaculum.
    Median nerve is the major component, which is compressed in carpal tunnel syndrome.

31. **A-T, B-T, C-T, D-T, E-F**

32. **A-T, B-T, C-T, D-F, E-F**
    Ossification is clockwise from capitate. Capitate and hamate—1, triquetrum—2 , lunate—3, scaphoid—4, trapezium—5, trapezoid—6, pisiform—12

33. **A-T, B-F, C-T, D-F, E-T**
    Most common sesamoid in hand is seen in flexor pollicis brevis tendon.The OS radiale externum is seen adjacent to the radial styloid in abductor pollicis longus. Bone age is assessed using left hand X-rays.

34. **A-T, B-T, C-F, D-T, E-F**
    Elbow is pivotal joint. Acromioclavicular is a complex synovial joint.

35. **A-F, B-T, C-T, D-F, E-T**
    There are six compartments in the extensor aspect of the wrist, beginning from the radial side.
    There is one tendon sheath in each compartment.
    1—extensor pollicis brevis, abductor pollicis longus, 2—extensor carpi radialis longus and brevis, 3—extensor pollicis longus, 4— extensor digitorum, 5—extensor digiti minimi, 6—extensor carpi ulnaris.

36. **A-T, B-F, C-F, D-F, E-F**
    De quervains tenosynovitis affects the first compartment, which has the extensor and abductor pollicis longus.It is common in

females and bilateral in 30%. The pain is over the radial styloid. The mechanism is due to wrist grip and ulnar deviation which causes angulation of the abductor pollicis longus and extensor carpi radialis longus against the radial styloid.

37. **A-T, B-T, C-T, D-F, E-T**

    Pregnancy and menopause are physiological states producing carpal tunnel syndrome. Occupational activities can cause.

    Accessory abductor digiti minimi produces ulnar nerve compression and accessory flexor digitorum superficialis produces median nerve compression. Wrist fracture, rheumatoid, diabetes, myxedema, alcoholism, acromegaly, gout, renal failure, hemodialysis, amyloidosis, obesit, OC pills are other causes.

38. **A-T, B-T, C-T, D-F, E-F**

    High signal is seen along the median nerve within the tunnel due to edema. This correlates with the edema seen in surgery. It is called pseudoganglion.

39. **A-T, B-F, C-T, D-T, E-F**

    Carpal tunnel syndrome is diagnosed by clinical examination and nerve conduction studies. High signal intensity in median nerve is not specific and can be seen even in asymptomatic and post-operative patients. Further high signal in seen in fat suppressed images. Atrophy is seen in the thenar eminence made by abductor pollicis brevis and opponens pollicis.

40. **A-T, B-F, C-T, D-T, E-T**

    MRI has a doubtful role in preoperative evaluation since diagnosis is based on clinical and nerve studies and treatment is same for all etiologies, conservative followed by resection of retinaculum. 20% have persistent symptoms, may be due to incomplete resection of retinaculum/scarring or tenosynovitis and MRI is useful in evaluation of these. Enhancement may be absent when wrist are held in extension or flexion. Tinel's and Phalen's are other clinical signs of carpal tunnel syndrome.

41. **A-T, B-T, C-T, D-T, E-F**

    Ganglions are either due to myxomatous degeneration of peri-articular connective tissue or remodelling of fibrous joint capsule or coalesence of synovial herniations. Common in 25-45 years. They have a fibrous capsule and filled with mucin.

    They have low signal in T1 and high signal in T2 and do not enhance.

42. **A-T, B-T,C-F, D-F, E-T**

    There are septations inside the ganglion. Intraosseous ganglion is common in the carpal bones and have similar signal intensity in

MRI. They are common in the subchondral bone, eccentric, well-defined with sclerotic rim.

43. **A-T, B-F, C-T, D-F, E-T**
It is seen in males, 20-40 years old. It is typically associated in those with negative ulnar variance, but can also be seen in those with neutral variance and positive ulnar variance.

44. **A-T, B-F, C-T, D-T, E-T**
Lichtman staging of Kienböck's disease
I—X-rays are normal, except for occasional compression fractures
II—sclerosis of lunate
III—collapse, A—no scapholunate dissociation, B—scapholunate dissociation.
IV—secondary osteoarthritis
Synovitis is seen in late stages.

45. **A-F, B-T, C-T, D-T, E-F**
Hyperparathyroidism, renal failure, crystal deposition disease, gout, sepsis are other causes.

46. **A-F, B-F, C-T, D-T, E-T**
Superficial bursae in the body are not present at birth and develop later due to movement and activity. Deep bursae are present at birth. Olecranin bursitis (Miner's, students elbow) is the most common superficial bursitis in the body. It can be secondary to infection in 20%, Staphylococcus aureus infection being the most common organism. In rheumatoid arthritis, can communicate with the elbow joint or rupture in the forearm.

7 Knee

1. **Anatomy of knee:**
   A. The outer two thirds of the menisci are avascular
   B. The posterior segment of the menisci are large than anterior segment
   C. Discoid meniscus is more common in the medial meniscus
   D. Lateral meniscus is firmly attached to capsule
   E. Medial meniscus is larger than the lateral meniscus

2. **Anatomy of the knee:**
   A. Lateral meniscus is attached to the capsule by superior and inferior meniscocapsular fascicles
   B. Normal meniscus shows low signal on T1 and high signal on T2 weighted images
   C. Intermeniscal ligament connects the posterior horns of the menisci
   D. The ligaments of Humphrey and Wrisberg extend from the posterior horn of the lateral meniscus to the medial femoral condyle
   E. Meniscomeniscal ligament connects the anterior horns of the menisci

3. **Knee joint:**
   A. The knee joint is a combination of condylar and saddle joints
   B. The knee joint is a modified hinge joint
   C. The three components of the knee joint are continuous
   D. The tibiofemoral space is 3 mm atleast
   E. Patellofemoral joint space is atleast 5 mm

4. **Knee joint capsule:**
   A. The tibial tuberosity is outside the capsule
   B. Coronary ligament tethers the medial meniscus to the medial tibial condyle
   C. Oblique popliteal ligament strengthens the posterior aspect of the capsule

    D. The lateral part of the capsule blends with the lateral collateral ligament

    E. Posteromedially the popliteus pierces the capsule

5. **The knee joint communicates with the following bursae:**
   - **A.** Medial gastrocnemius-semimembranous
   - **B.** Prepatellar
   - **C.** Infrapatellar
   - **D.** Lateral gastrocnemius
   - **E.** Popliteus

6. **Knee:**
   - **A.** Skyline view of the patella is taken with the knee flexed
   - **B.** Tunnel view is useful for loose body evaluation
   - **C.** Meniscal abnormalities are best seen in T1W images
   - **D.** Patellofemoral joint is best assessed in the sagittal images
   - **E.** Most common cause of lipohemarthrosis is tibial plateau fractures

7. **Pigmented villonodular synovitis in knee:**
   - **A.** Most common site for the disease
   - **B.** Usually associated with erosion of the articular cortices
   - **C.** Produces a slight reduction in size of the articular cavity
   - **D.** Can be diagnosed by double contrast arthography in almost all cases
   - **E.** Avascular on angiography

8. **Discoid meniscus:**
   - **A.** Is very prone for tear
   - **B.** Common in the medial meniscus
   - **C.** Diagnosed only if seen in atleast five contiguous images
   - **D.** 12% incidence
   - **E.** Asymptomatic

9. **Knee synovium:**
   - **A.** The synovium covers the meniscus
   - **B.** Synovium lines the capsule
   - **C.** Lines suprapatellar bursa
   - **D.** Lines patellar tendon
   - **E.** Covers the anterior and not posterior cruciate ligament

10. **Knee joint:**
    - **A.** Oblique popliteal ligament is an expansion of semimembranosus
    - **B.** Anterior cruciate is attached to the medial femoral condyle
    - **C.** PCL is shorter than ACL
    - **D.** There is a bursa between the cruciate ligaments
    - **E.** Both cruciate ligaments are taut in every position of the joint

11. **Knee:**
    A. Humphrey's ligament passes anterior to the ACL
    B. Wrisberg's ligament passes posterior to PCL
    C. Meniscofemoral ligament attaches the posterior horn of medial meniscus to the lateral condyle
    D. Lateral meniscus forms a near complete ring
    E. Lateral meniscus is larger

12. **Movements of knee joint and the causative muscles:**
    A. Flexion—biceps
    B. Extension—quadriceps
    C. Unlocking flexed knee—popliteus
    D. Medial rotation—biceps
    E. Lateral rotation—popliteus

13. **Intercondylar area:**
    A. The anterior cruciate ligament is the most anterior structure
    B. The posterior cruciate ligament is the most posterior structure
    C. The posterior horn of medial meniscus is attached just behind the intercondylar eminence
    D. The anterior and posterior horns of lateral meniscus are attached respectively anterior and posterior to the intercondylar eminence
    E. The anterior horn of medial meniscus is situated posterior to the anterior horn of lateral meniscus

14. **Meniscal tear:**
    A. Meniscal tear always involves atleast one articular surface
    B. Radial tears are along the long axis of meniscus
    C. Longitudinal tears are perpendicular to the long axis of the meniscus
    D. Bucket handle tear happens when an extensive longitudinal tear results in separation of inner portion of meniscus into the notch
    E. Peripheral tears heal with conservative management

15. **Knee:**
    A. The patellar apex is 1 cm above the the knee joint
    B. The patella has a large medial facet and small large facet
    C. Fabella is the sesamoid in the lateral head of gastrocnemius
    D. The lateral condyle bears the majority of the patellar articulation
    E. The medial femoral condyle is larger than the lateral condyle

16. **Bipartite patella:**
    A. Most common in the supramedial portion of the patella
    B. Features of bipartite patella are specific and differentiates it from fracture
    C. They are usually bilateral
    D. Horizontal
    E. Normal ossification centers of patella appear at 1 year

17. **Muscles and their origin:**
    A. Tensor fascia lata—anterior inferior iliac spine
    B. Rectus femoris reflected head—acetabulum
    C. Vastus lateralis—greater trochanter
    D. Vastus medialis—femoral shaft
    E. Adductor longus—pubic rami

18. **Muscles and insertion:**
    A. Gracilis—medial tibial condyle
    B. Vastus intermedius—patella
    C. Tensor fascia lata—iliotibial tract
    D. Adductor longus—linea aspera
    E. Sartorius—medial tibial condyle

19. **Muscles and their insertion:**
    A. Biceps femoris—head of fibula
    B. Semitendinosus—lateral femoral condyle
    C. Adductor brevis—lesser trochanter
    D. Adductor magnus—adductor tubercle
    E. Vastus medius—patella

20. **Meniscal tear:**
    A. Double PCL sign is an indicator of bucket handle tear
    B. Meniscocapsular separation is common in medial meniscus
    C. Septations are seen in meniscal cysts
    D. High signal in a meniscus after surgery indicates recurrence
    E. MR arthrography is the best modality for diagnosing recurrent or new tear in a postsurgical patient

21. **Anatomy of knee joint:**
    A. Articular cartilage has low signal in T1
    B. Hyaline articular cartilage is seen in the trochlear groove of the distal femur and dorsal surface of the patella
    C. STIR sequence is the best for assessment of hyaline cartilages
    D. The trabecular bone in the distal femur is stronger than the cortical bone
    E. The subchondral plate absorbs the dynamic stresses near the knee joint

22. **Bone contusions:**
    A. Bone contusions are best seen on T2W sequence
    B. Contusion in ACL injury is seen in lateral femoral condyle and lateral tibial plateau
    C. Contusion in patellar dislocation is seen in the anterolateral aspect of lateral femoral condyle
    D. Osteochondritis dissecans is seen in the medial aspect of lateral femoral condyle
    E. Fracture line is seen as a low signal only in STIR images

23. **Signs of instability in osteochondritis dissecans are:**
    A. Best assessed in T1W images
    B. Linear high signal intensity around the fragment
    C. High signal intensity in linear defect in the overlying cartilage
    D. Cystic changes >5 mm between the fragment and the host bone
    E. A focal defect in cartilage, > 5 mm

24. **Anatomy of cruciate ligaments:**
    A. The ACL is seen medial PCL
    B. The ACL is more homogeneous than PCL
    C. ACL prevents posterior translation of tibia relative to femur
    D. ACL is seen as a taut structure parallel to intercondylar roof
    E. PCL is seen as an arching structure medially

25. **Collateral ligaments:**
    A. The superficial part of medial collateral ligament extends 7 cm inferior to the joint line
    B. The deeper aspect of medial collateral ligament is called as medial capsular ligament
    C. Tibial collateral bursa is seen between the superficial and deeper layers of medial collateral ligament
    D. Collateral ligaments show low signal in all sequences
    E. Biceps femoris is a part of the lateral stabilizing complex

26. **Cruciate ligament injuries:**
    A. ACL injury is caused by twisting injury due to internal rotation of the femur on a fixed tibia, combined with a valgus stress
    B. Empty notch sign in coronal image is a sign of ACL injury
    C. Contusion in the anterior portions of distal femur and tibial plateau
    D. Deepening of sulcus terminalis in the lateral femoral condyle
    E. Chronically torn ACL may appear normal

27. **Knee arthrography:**
    A. Medial meniscus is more commonly damaged in younger patients

B. Double contrast is not as good as single contrast arthrogram for diagnosis of cruciate tears
C. Filling of gastrocnemius bursa occurs in 2/3rd of cases
D. Anterior tears are confused with prepatellar fat pad
E. Lateral tear may be confused with the popliteal bursa

28. **Meniscal cyst:**
    A. Parameniscal cyst is more common in the lateral side
    B. Normal meniscus should be seen in three contiguous sagittal images
    C. In discoid meniscus, meniscus seen in more than 2 contiguous images
    D. The posterior horn of the lateral meniscus is the largest meniscus structure
    E. Meniscal cyst is not seen without meniscal tear

29. **Meniscal cyst:**
    A. Lateral meniscal cyst can be palpated clinically
    B. Medial meniscal cyst can be seen in Hoffa's pad of fat anteriorly
    C. Cysts in the posterior most aspect of medial meniscus are not accessible during meniscectomy
    D. T2W sagittal images are best for midmeniscal cysts
    E. Produced due to mucoid production by synovial cells in meniscus

30. **Causes of meniscal cyst:**
    A. Trauma
    B. Neoplastic
    C. Abnormal cartilage metabolism
    D. Infection
    E. Haemorrhage

31. **Patellar tendinitis:**
    A. Seen in distal third of the tendon close to the insertion
    B. Best seen in sagittal images
    C. More in the anterior aspect of the tendon
    D. High signal in peritendinous area in acute stage
    E. Tendon is thickened in chronic stage

32. **Common causes of bilateral patellar tendon rupture:**
    A. Trauma
    B. Diabetes
    C. Hyperparathyroidism
    D. Rheumatoid arthritis
    E. Transient patellar dislocation

33. **Transient patellar dislocation:**
    A. Associated with lateral meniscal tear
    B. Major ligamental injury is associated in 30%
    C. Due to external rotation of femur
    D. Most common cause of hemoarthrosis in young conscripts
    E. Seen in old inactive people

34. **Transient patellar dislocation:**
    A. Increased signal intensity in the lateral patellar retinaculum
    B. Dislocation is common on the medial aspect
    C. The patella is tilted laterally
    D. Contusion is seen in the medial femoral condyle
    E. Contusion is seen in the medial articular surface of the patella

35. **True patellar dislocation:**
    A. Posterior dislocation is the most common
    B. Anterior dislocation is due to violent hyperextension
    C. Popliteal artery injury is more common in posterior dislocation than anterior dislocation
    D. Rotational dislocation is the most rare type of dislocation
    E. Extensor mechanism disruption is seen in posterior dislocation

36. **Dislocation of patella:**
    A. Rotatory dislocation is associated with severe ligamentous injuries
    B. O Donoghues triad has injury to ACL, lateral meniscus and lateral retinaculum
    C. In AP view, there is lateral displacement of tibial plateau more than 1/4th of condylar width
    D. The unhappy triad is due to valgus stress
    E. Fractures in knees are not usually associated with dislocation

37. **Associations of chondromalacia patellae:**
    A. Rheumatoid arthritis
    B. Menisectomy
    C. Immobilisation
    D. Fracture
    E. Hemarthrosis

38. **Radiological differential diagnosis for Baker's cysts:**
    A. Popliteal artery aneurysm
    B. Tear of gastrocnemius
    C. Liposarcoma
    D. Ganglion
    E. Simple bone cyst

39. **Grading of chondromalacia patella:**
    A. Absence of cartilage is grade 4 in arthroscopy
    B. MRI is very useful for grade 1 and 2 lesions
    C. Arthroscopy is 100% sensitive and specific for grade 4 lesions
    D. Focal low signal region is the earliest sign of chondromalacia
    E. Gradient echo images better than double echo spin echo images for assessment

40. **Patella:**
    A. Patella alta is highly placed patella
    B. Patella baja is low position of patella
    C. Patella adentro—lateral subluxation of patella
    D. Patella baja associated with Osgood-Schlatter disease
    E. Patella baja—patella placed below the level of femoral trochlear groove

41. **Patellar dislocation:**
    A. Injury to medial patellofemoral ligament always requires surgery
    B. Presence of osteochondral fragment requires arthroscopic evaluation
    C. Loose body requires arthroscopy
    D. Bone contusion requires only conservative treatment
    E. Recurrent dislocation seen in 50-65% of initial trauma cases

42. **Patella alta:**
    A. Causes patellofemoral joint instability
    B. Association with chondromalacia patella
    C. More common in women
    D. Increased incidence of patellar dislocation
    E. Axial images are best for assessment of patella alta

43. **Patella alta is associated with:**
    A. Osgood-Schlatter disease
    B. Sinding-Larsen-Johansson disease
    C. Quardriceps tear
    D. Patellar subluxation
    E. Joint effusion

44. **Patella baja is associated with:**
    A. Quadriceps rupture
    B. Achondroplasia
    C. Postsurgical
    D. Osgood-Schlatter disease
    E. Homocystinuria

45. **Baker's cyst is associated with:**
    A. Haemophilia
    B. Sarcoidosis
    C. Pigmented villonodular synovitis
    D. Meniscal tear
    E. Hypothyroidism

46. **Baker's cyst:**
    A. Rheumatoid arthritis is the most common arthritis associated with Baker's cyst
    B. The cyst formation has a direct correlation with the severity of the osteoarthritis
    C. Lateral meniscal tear is the most common meniscal injury associated
    D. Ultrasound is more sensitive than arthrography
    E. MRI is the best imaging modality for diagnosis

47. **Baker's cyst:**
    A. Seen between gastrocnemius and semitendinosus bursa
    B. Gadolinium administration shows enhancement of the cyst wall
    C. Doppler shows peripheral flow within the cyst
    D. DVT is the most common complication of Baker's cyst
    E. Increased risk of DVT with Baker's cyst

48. **Complications of Baker's cyst are:**
    A. Infection
    B. Haemorrhage
    C. DVT
    D. Sarcoma
    E. Posterior compartment syndrome

49. **Baker's cyst:**
    A. There is two way flow of fluid between the cyst and the joint
    B. Lined by synovium
    C. Primary cysts show high viscosity fluid
    D. In Bunsen valve type the neck is compressed by enlarging cyst
    E. Can be seen between lateral head of gastrocnemius and biceps

ANSWERS

1. **A-F, B-T, C-F, D-F, E-T**

   Menisci are fibrocartilagenous discs found in the knee joint. The medial meniscus is larger than the lateral meniscus. Each meniscus has an anterior horn, posterior horn and a body. The outer third of meniscus is well vascularised and the inner third is avascular. The medial meniscus is firmly attached to the knee joint capsule throughout its course. The lateral meniscus is less firmly attached to the capsule. It is attached at the posterior aspect by the superior and inferior meniscocapsular fascicles, at the level of popliteus tendon. Discoid meniscus, an anatomical variant, is commonly seen in the lateral side.

2. **A-T, B-F, C-F, D-T, E-F**

   The menisci have low signal in all the MRI sequences. The transverse, intermeniscal ligament connects the anterior horns of both the menisci. The oblique meniscomeniscal ligament connects the posterior horn of one meniscus to the anterior horn of the other meniscus. The meniscofemoral ligaments of Humphrey and Wrisberg connect the posterior horn of the lateral meniscus to the medial femoral condyle and are seen adjacent to the anterior and posterior margins of posterior cruciate ligaments.

3. **A-T, B-T, C-T, D-T, E-F**

   Knee is a complex synovial hinge joint, with two condylar joints in between the femoral and tibial articular surfaces and a saddle between patella and femur.

   Tibiofemoral joint space and patellofemoral joint space measure at least 3 mm.

4. **A-F, B-T, C-T, D-F, E-F**

   Tibial tuberosity is included within the capsule, which is attached superiorly to the intercondylar fossa and margins of patella and inferiorly to include the tibial condyles.

   The lateral part of the capsule does not blend with the lateral collateral ligament, unlike the medial aspect which blends with the medial collateral ligament. The popliteus pierces the posterolateral aspect of the capsule.

5. **A-T, B-T, C-F, D-F, E-T**

   Knee joint communicates with medial gastrocnemius (in 50%), lateral gastrocnemius, suprapatellar and popliteus. Does not communicate with infrapatellar, superficial and deep prepatellar and biceps bursae.

6. **A-T, B-T, C-T, D-F, E-T**

   Skyline view is essential for evaluation of patellar lesions. Tunnel view focuses on the intercondylar notch and useful for loose bodies Patellofemoral joint is best assessed in axial images.

7. **A-T, B-T, C-T, D-T, E-F**

   Hypervascular in angiography. The joint size increases initially and narrows in later stages. Low signal seen inT1 and T2W MRI.

8. **A-T, B-F, C-T, D-F, E-F**

   Diagnosed if there is continuity between the anterior and posterior third of the meniscus, in at least five contiguous 3 mm images. This is often symptomatic. Commonly seen in lateral meniscus. 1.5-3% incidence, 15% in Asia, 01.-0.3% in medial meniscus.

9. **A-F, B-T, C-T, D-F, E-F**

   The meniscal surfaces and suprapatellar bursa are not lined by meniscus. The infrapatellar pad of fat separates the synovium and patellar tendon. Both the cruciate ligaments are covered by meniscus.

10. **A-T, B-F, C-T, D-T, E-T**

    Anterior cruciate ligament—from anterior tibial intercondylar area—medial part of lateral femoral condyle. Prevents femur moving backwards on tibia. Posterior cruciate ligament—from posterior tibial intercondylar area-lateral part of medial femoral condyle. Prevents posterior sliding of tibia on femur. PCL is stronger and shorter than ACL.

11. **A-F, B-T, C-F, D-T, E-F**

    Meniscofemoral ligament passes from the posterior horn of the lateral meniscus to the medial femoral condyle. This divides into two and when passing anterior to PCL, it is called the Humphrey's ligament and, when posterior to PCL is called Wrisberg's ligament. Medial meniscus is larger.

12. **A-T, B-T, C-T, D-F, E-F**

    Medial rotation of flexed knee is by popliteus, semimembranosus and semitendinosus.
    Lateral rotation of flexed knee is by biceps femoris. Flexion is also helped by semitendinosus and semimembranosus.

13. **A-F, B-T, C-F, D-T, E-F**

    From anterior to posterior, the structures attached to the inter-condylar area are:
    Anterior horn of medial meniscus, anterior cruciate ligament, anterior horn of lateral meniscus, posterior horn of lateral meniscus, posterior horn of medial meniscus and posterior cruciate ligament.

14. **A-T, B-F, C-F, D-T, E-T**
Meniscal tears are either due to trauma or degeneration. It can be vertical or horizontal. Vertical tears can be: 1) Longitudinal—along the long axis of the meniscus and 2) Radial—perpendicular to the long axis of the meniscus. Horizontal tear extends through the substance of meniscus, parallel to the tibial plateau dividing it into superior and inferior portions. With extensive longitudinal tear, the inner portion of the meniscus, displaces into notch resulting in bucket handle tear. Tear occurring in the outer third of the meniscus is called peripheral tear and it heals with conservative management, since this portion of meniscus has a good vascular supply. Tears in inner third of meniscus require debridement or partial meniscectomy.

15. **A-T, B-F, C-T, D-T, E-T**
Patella has a large lateral facet and a smaller medial facet.

16. **A-F, B-F, C-T, D-T, E-F**
It is due to failure of fusion of patellar ossification centers, which normally appear at 3-6 years and fuse. Seen as a oblique cleft in the supralateral margin of the patella. Occasionally, may be horizontal.

17. **A-F, B-T, C-T, D-F, E-F**

18. **A-F, B-T, C-T, D-T, E-T**

19. **A-T, B-F, C-T, D-T, E-T**
Muscles—origins and insertions
Tensor fascia lata—anterior superior iliac spine—iliotibial band
Rectus femoris—straight head—anterior inferior iliac spine—patella
Reflected head—acetabulum, hip joint capsule
Sartorius—ASIS—medial tibial condyle
Vastus intermedius—femoral shaft—patella
Vastus medius—greater trochanter, linea aspera—medial patella
Vastus lateralis—greater trochanter—iliotibial tract
Gracilis—body and inferior ramus of pubis—medial tibia
Pectineus—pectin pubis—lesster trochanter and linea aspera
Adductor longus—body of pubis—linea aspera
Adductor brevis—inferior ramus and body of pubis—lesser trochanter, linea aspera
Adductor magnus—inferior pubic ramus and ischial ramus—linea, aspera, adductor tubercle.
Semimembranosus—ischial tuberosity—lateral femoral condyle
Semitendinosus—ischial tuberosity—medial surface of tibia
Bicep femoris—long head—ischial tuberosity
Short head—linea aspera—head of fibula

20. **A-T, B-T, C-T, D-F, E-T**

Meniscal tear is seen as abnormal high signal intensity that communicates with one of both articular surfaces. Some tears have only altered morphology such as absence of a portion of meniscus, marginal irregularity or a focal defect. Bucket handle tear is seen as a double PCL sign, on sagittal images. Blunting of the free edge of the meniscus or a displaced fragment within the intercondylar notch is seen in coronal images. Meniscocapsular separation, common in the medial meniscus, is suggested by fluid tracking between meniscus and adjacent capsule. Meniscal cysts occur due to extrusion of synovial fluid through a horizontal tear, collecting at meniscocapsular interface and have fluid signal with septations. After surgery, the meniscus may be absent or may appear normal. Abnormal high signal may persist after a tear has healed and so it does not reliably predict the presence of a new or recurrent tear. MR arthrography will confirm recurrence, if contrast extends into the meniscus.

21. **A-T, B-T, C-T, D-T, E-F**

The knee is a hinge joint. The subchondral plate is the thin layer of cortical bone along the articular surfaces, which provides support for the overlying cartilage. The underlying trabecular bone, composed of many osseus struts, is very stronger than the cortical bone and plays a very important role in absorbing dynamic stresses near joints by dissipating axial forces from the subchondral plate and articular cartilage. Hyaline cartilage is present along the medial and lateral condyles and trochlear groove of the distal femur and dorsal surface of the patella. The cartilage is hypo on T2 and hyper on T2 sequences. STIR is the best sequence for evaluation of cartilage sequences, since it gives an excellent contrast between the high signal of fluid within the joint and low signal of the cartilage.

22. **A-F, B-T, C-T, D-T, E-F**

Bone contusions or bruises or microtrabecular fractures are trabecular injuries resulting from impaction forces as is associated with hemorrhage and edema. STIR and fat suppressed T2W sequences are the best, where the contusions are seen as poorly defined focal high signal areas. They are missed easily in T2W sequences without fat suppression. Radiographically occult fractures are seen as linear focus of low signal intensity on T1W images and high or low signal intensity on STIR images. In anterior cruciate ligament, the contusion is seen in the lateral femoral condyle and posterolateral tibial plateau. In lateral patellar dislocation, it is seen in the antero-lateral margin of the lateral femoral condyle. In osteochondritis dissecans, it is seen in the medial aspect of the lateral femoral condyle.

23. **A-F, B-T, C-T, D-T, E-T**
Osteochondritis dissecans
High signal intensity line between fragment and parent bone indicates fluid/granulation tissue. This is not an infallible sign. Fluid encircling fragment, focal cystic areas beneath fragment, high signal through cartilage, focal defect are more reliable. Enhancement of zone between fragment and parent indicates instability. Best assessed by T2W images.

24. **A-F, B-F, C-F, D-T, E-T**
Cruciate ligaments lie within the intercondylar notch. The anterior cruciate ligament is found laterally. It is seen as a low signal band, which may contain higher signal intensity areas due to collageneous structure. The anterior margin is taut and parallel to intercondylar roof. The posterior cruciate ligament lies within the medial notch and is an arching, low signal intensity band, which is more homogeneous than ACL. The ACL prevents the anterior translation of tibia over femur and PCL prevents the posterior translation of tibia relative to femur.

25. **A-T, B-T, C-T, D-T, E-T**
Collateral ligaments are seen as low signal structures in all sequences. The medial collateral ligament has a superficial and deep layer. The superficial fibers extend from the medial aspect of the medial femoral condyle to the medial tibia approximately 7 cm inferior to the joint line. The deep component, medial capsular ligament is attached to the medial meniscus. The tibial collateral bursa lies between these two layers. The lateral ligamentous complex includes from lateral to medial, illiotibial band, lateral capsular ligament—meniscotibial and meniscofemoral ligament, lateral collateral ligament, biceps femoris tendon and popliteus tendon. The collateral ligaments are best seen in coronal images.

26. **A-F, B-T, C-T, D-T, E-T**
ACL is injured by a twisting injury due to external rotation of the femur on a fixed tibia, combined with a valgus stress. The signs are; Direct: 1—disruption of ligament; 2—irregular contour to ligament; 3—high signal within ligament; 4—empty notch in coronal images; Indirect: 1—contusion in the lateral femoral condyle and lateral posterolateral tibial plateau, (rotational injury); 2—contusion in anterior portions of distal femur and tibial plateau (hyperextension injury); 3—deepening of sulcus terminalis in lateral femoral condyle; 4—segond fracture of lateral tibial plateau;

5—MRI anterior drawer sign; 6-buckling of PCL. Chronic ACL tear: 1—focal angulation of the ligament, 2—fragmentation 3—non-visualisation of ligament, but no edema, 4—normal appearance due to bridging scar.

27. **A-T, B-F, C-T, D-T, E-T**
Double contrast arthrogram uses air and is as good as single contrast arthrogram. MR arthrogram has replaced conventional arthrograms.

28. **A-T, B-F, C-T, D-F, E-F**
Normal meniscus should be seen in 2 contiguous sagittal images. If seen in more than 2, it is discoid meniscus and in less than 2, it is a meniscal tear. The posterior horn of the medial meniscus is the largest horn. The other horns are equal sized.

29. **A-T, B-T, C-T, D-T, E-T**
Lateral meniscus cyst is easily palpated, because it is loosely attached to joint structures. The medial meniscus cyst, expands through ligaments, either anteriorly or posteriorly and settles in a place far from the site of origin, making palpation difficult. Posterior aspect of medial meniscus is a blind area during meniscectomy. T2W coronal images are the best for assessing mid-meniscus.

30. **A-T, B-F, C-T, D-T, E-T**
Torn meniscus is a common cause. Associated with horizontal clevage tears. Believed to arise due to leakage of synovial fluid through torn meniscus/compression injury of peripheral aspect of degenerate meniscus.

31. **A-F, B-F, C-F, D-T, E-T**
The proximal part of tendon is commonly involved. The posterior aspect of the tendon is affected earlier. Axial images are best for diagnosing. In acute stage, the high signal is seen in peritendinous area and associated with subcutaneous edema. This lasts for 2 weeks. In chronic stage, the tendon is thickened and shows high signal, which is due to tenocyte hyperplasia/angiogenesis/loss of collagen architecture/micro tears.

32. **A-F, B-T, C-T, D-T, E-F**
Bilateral patellar tendon rupture requires underlying diseases like rheumatoid, hyperparathyroidism or diabetes mellitus.

33. **A-F, B-T, C-F, D-T, E-F**
Associated with medial meniscal tear. It is common in young active people.

The mechanism is an attempt to slow forward translation, with medial pivoting on a planted foot, thereby producing internal rotation of femur and quadriceps rotation.

34. **A-F, B-F, C-T, D-F, E-T**
There is disruption or increased signal intensity in the medial patellar retinaculum, with lateral tilt of the patella. Increased signal is seen in the nonarticular surface of the lateral femoral condyle and medial articular surface of the patella.

35. **A-F, B-T, C-F, D-T, E-T**
Dislocation is mentioned in terms of relation of position of tibia with femur.
Anterior—most common, violent hyperextension force, injury to popliteal artery, peroneal nerve.
Posterior—direct blow, no arterial injury, extensor mechanism disrupted.
Rotatory, medial and lateral are rare.

36. **A-T, B-F, C-F, D-T, E-T**
The unhappy triad is due to valgus stress and has ACL, medial meniscus and medial retinaculum injury. In rotatory dislocation, the dislocation is mild and in AP view of knee there will be lateral dislocation of the tibia in relation to femur, but only less than 1/4th of condyle width.

37. **A-F, B-T, C-T, D-T, E-T**
Chondromalacia is softening of patellar cartilage. Idiopathic, blunt trauma, ochronosis, chondrocalcinosis, gout, aging and surgical shaving are other causes.

38. **A-T, B-T, C-T, D-T, E-F**
Cystic adventitial degeneration of popliteal A (Erdheim mucoid degeneration), nerve, sheath tumours, myxoid tumours, meniscal cyst are other differentials.

39. **A-T, B-T, C-T, D-T, E-F**
Arthroscopic grading of chondromalacia patellae.
1—minimal change with no break in articular surface
2—areas of fibrillation or fissuring, with irregular, rough surface
3—fibrillation and fissuring extending to subchondral bone (crabmeat appearance)
4—absence of articular cartilage, with exposed subchondral bone
MRI staging based on grade, size, location, degree of flexion and sclerosis.
I—intact surface, thickening or high signal in cartilage, <10 mm
II—irregular surface without complete cartilage loss, 10-25 mm

III—full thickness loss of cartilage. Contact of joint fluid with bone, >25mm
MRI is very useful in early stages, where arthroscopy is unnecessary since there is no arthroscopic treatment. Double echo SE images are the best.

40. **A-T, B-T, C-F, D-T, E-T**
In patella baja, the patella is unusually placed below the level of femoral trochlear groove. It is also seen in patellar realignment surgeries. Patella adentro is medial subluxation of patella.

41. **A-T, B-T, C-T, D-T, E-T**
Patellar dislocation more common in the lateral side.

42. **A-T, B-T, C-T, D-T, D-T**
In axial images, the normal patellas inferior pole is seen at the level of superior aspect of femoral trochlear groove. In alta, it is situated far above this level and in baja, below this level.

43. **A-T, B-T, C-F, D-T, E-T**
Patella alta refers to superior displacement of the patella. It is measured by the Insall Salvati ratio, which is a ratio of the maximum diagonal length of patella to the length of patellar tendon. Normal ratio is 1:1. If patellar tendon length is longer, it is called patella alta. It is associated with patellar tendon rupture, patellar subluxation/dislocation, Osgood-Schlatter, Sinding-Larsen disease, joint effusion, chondromalacia patellae, homocystinuria, neuromuscular disease and patellar sleeve fracture.

44. **A-T, B-T, C-T, D-T, E-F**
Patella baja is inferior displacement of patella and is diagnosed when, the patellar length is more than the patellar tendon length. The common causes are quadriceps tear, Osgood Schlatter disease, achondroplasia, neuromuscular disease and surgical transfer of the tibial tubercle.

45. **A-T, B-T, C-T, D-T, E-T**
Osteoarthritis, rheumatoid arthritis, gout, Reiter's disease, psoriasis, SLE, infection and other knee ligament tears are also associated. The most common mechanism of formation is synovial proliferation with effusion.

46. **A-F, B-T, C-F, D-F, E-T**
There is high prevalence of Baker's cyst in rheumatoid arthritis, but osteoarthritis is the more common arthritis and many Baker's cysts are associated with osteoarthritis. Posterior horn of medial meniscus is the most commonly injured meniscus. Arthrography is more sensitive than ultrasound.

47. **A-F, B-T, C-F, D-F, E-T**
    Seen between the medial head of gastrocnemius and semimembranosus. In inflammatory arthritis, there is enhancement of the synovium and cyst wall. Doppler does not show any flow and is seen if there is aneurysm. Pseudothrombophlebitis is the most common complication.

48. **A-T, B-T, C-T, D-F, E-T**
    Pseudothrombophlebitis due to leaking of fluid into gastrocnemius producing symptoms of DVT and pulmonary embolism are other complications.

49. **A-F, B-T, C-T, D-T, E-T**
    There is valve at the site of communication between the cyst and the joint, which allows flow only from the joint into the cyst. In Bunsen type of valve, the enlarging cyst exerts pressure on the opening. Primary cysts show high viscosity and have synovial folds, scarring and membranes which produce the valves. Secondary cysts are due to arthritis. The supralateral type is seen between the lateral head of gastrocnemius and biceps and the popliteal type is anterior, the popliteus and beneath the lateral meniscus.

8

Spine and Hip

1. **Anterior scalloping in vertebra is seen in:**
   A. Lymphoma
   B. CA cervix metastasis
   C. Tuberculosis
   D. Down's syndrome
   E. Ankylosing spondylitis

2. **Vertebra:**
   A. There are 31 vertebrae
   B. There are 33 pairs of spinal nerves
   C. Spinal cord is well resolved in CT scans, in the upper cervical region
   D. CT myelography is preferred to simple CT for evaluating intradural structures in the lumbar region.
   E. Complete rupture of posterior longitudinal ligament alone is sufficient for causing instability

3. **Normal density values of the following structures:**
   A. Spinal cord—35-70 HU
   B. Intervertebral disc—50-100 HU
   C. Dural sac—5-25 HU
   D. CSF—10-20 HU
   E. Fat—60-100 HU

4. **The following are contrast enhancing structures in CT scan:**
   A. Dorsal root ganglia   B. Meninges
   C. Nerve roots   D. Spinal cord
   E. Intervertebral disc

5. **Contrast enhancing structures in MRI scan:**
   A. Dorsal root ganglia
   B. Bone marrow
   C. Blood vessels
   D. Spinal cord
   E. Intervertebral disc

6. **MRI of spinal cord:**
   A. T2W MR images are better than CT myelographic images
   B. Disc changes are better visualized in T1W images
   C. The cancellous bone is hyperintense in T1W images in adults
   D. Fat suppression images are essential after contrast enhancement
   E. Gray and white matter can be differentiated in high resolution MR images

7. **Vertebral body:**
   A. The vertebral trabeculae are vertical only
   B. The superior articular facet faces anteriorly
   C. The inferior articular facet faces anteriorly
   D. The pars interarticularis is the portion of lamina between the articular facets
   E. The vertical trabeculae bear the weight

8. **Intervertebral disc:**
   A. The discs are thinnest in the lumbar region
   B. The discs are thickest anteriorly in the cervical and lumbar region
   C. The posterolateral aspects of the lumbar discs are not reinforced by posterior longitudinal ligaments
   D. The nerve fibres from vertebral nerves innervate the peripheral aspect of the nucleus pulposus
   E. The disc is vascular in the children

9. **Spinous ligaments:**
   A. The supraspinous ligament extends from axis to the sacrum
   B. There are three layers in anterior longitudinal ligament
   C. The basivertebral vein is situated between the PLL and the posterior vertebral body
   D. The PLL is attached to the dura
   E. The PLL shows a bulge, which is prominent in extension

10. **Intervertebral disc:**
    A. A secondary cartilaginous joint
    B. Made up of hyaline cartilage
    C. The nucleus pulposus is made of Type II collagen and proteoglycans
    D. The inner fibres of annulus pulposus insert into the hyaline cartilage
    E. The outer fibres of annulus pulposus insert beyond vertebral margins
    F. The annulus fibrosus has 80% of water

11. **Causes of wide disk spaces:**
    A. Sickle cell anemia
    B. Osteoporosis
    C. Acromegaly
    D. Gaucher's disease
    E. Hyperextension spinal injury

12. **Intervertebral canal:**
    A. The cervical canals are oriented posterolaterally
    B. The lumbar canals are oriented laterally
    C. Foraminal veins support the nerves in the cervical foramens instead of the fat
    D. The thoracic intervertebral canals are the smallest
    E. Oblique views are necessary for demonstrating cervical foramens

13. **Spinal nerve roots:**
    A. All the spinal nerve roots exit below the level of the pedicle
    B. If there is a disc prolapse between C7 and T1, the T1 nerve root will be compressed
    C. If there is a disc prolapse between C5 and C6, C6 root will be compressed
    D. If there is a disc prolapse between L3/4, the L3 root will be compressed
    E. Cervical root ganglia are easily identified than lumbar dorsal root ganglia

14. **Spinal nerve roots:**
    A. Sympathetic fibres are carried along with the dorsal nerve roots
    B. The thoracic nerve roots bend downwards and then upwards to exit through the foramen
    C. The lumbosacral roots exit below the level of intervertebral disc
    D. The sacral root may lie at different level in either side
    E. The root sheath above the level of conjoined nerve root is absent

15. **Important tendon jerks and their innervation:**
    A. Knee—L2,3,4
    B. Ankle—S2,3
    C. Supinator—C5,6
    D. Biceps—C5,6
    E. Triceps—C5,6

16. **Myelography:**
    A. The spine is flexed during lumbar puncture to increase the interspinous distance
    B. The cervical puncture is performed in prone position only
    C. The cisternal puncture is done in lateral decubitus position
    D. The iliac crest is at the level of L4
    E. The cervical subarachnoid space is capacious than the lumbar subarachnoid space

17. **Spinous ligaments:**
    A. PLL is attached to the posterior vertebral bodies
    B. ALL is firmly attached to the anterior aspect of the vertebral discs
    C. The ALL tapers inferiorly
    D. The PLL widens inferiorly
    E. The PLL continues superiorly as the tectal membrane

18. **Spinous ligaments:**
    A. The ligamentum flavum is very thick in the lumbar region
    B. The ligamentum flavum has the highest intensity among the spinous ligaments
    C. The ligamentum flavum has a 35% change in its dimension with flexion and extension
    D. The epidural fat is seen outside the ligamentum flavum, posteriorly
    E. The interspinous ligaments are well developed only in the lumbar region

19. **Vertebral joints:**
    A. The facet joints are synovial joints
    B. The inferior articular process is anterior to that of the superior articular process in the facet joint
    C. The facet joint is innervated by medial division of posterior primary ramus at the level below the joint
    D. The lumbar facet joints are the largest in the spine
    E. Menisci are present in lumbar facet joints

20. **Spine:**
    A. Ossification of posterior longitudinal ligament producer symptoms in age group later than degenerative disc disease
    B. OPLL always shows low signal in T1 and T2
    C. Herniated disk seen in 35% of normal population
    D. Scar enhancement occurs regardless of time since surgery
    E. Arachnoiditis enhances lesser than drop metastasis

21. **Vertebral muscles:**
    A. The flexor muscles are supplied by the posterior primary rami
    B. The extensor muscles are supplied by the anterior primary rami
    C. The psoas muscle is the major muscle controlling flexion of the lumbar spine
    D. Sternocleidomastoid is the major flexor of the cervical spine
    E. Erector spinae cause extension and rotation of spine

22. **Types of joints in vertebra:**
    A. Intervertebral joints—synovial
    B. Facet joints—synovial
    C. Luschka's joints—fibrous
    D. Joints between transverse processes—fibrous
    E. Joints between spinous processes—fibrous

23. **Causes of spinal cord atrophy:**
    A. Friedreich's ataxia
    B. AV malformations
    C. Cervical disc herniation
    D. Syringomyelia
    E. Amyotrophic lateral sclerosis

24. **Causes of narrow intervertebral foramen:**
    A. Meningomyelocele
    B. Klippel-Feil syndrome
    C. Posterior subluxation of cervical spine
    D. Diastomatomyelia
    E. Dural ectasices

25. **The following are contents of the intervertebral foramen:**
    A. Foraminal veins   B. Epidural fat
    C. Dorsal root ganglia   D. Nerve roots
    E. Lymphatics

26. **Vertebral blood supply:**
    A. The right intercostal artery supplies the right side of vertebra only
    B. The basivertebral veins are prominently seen in the cervical vertebra
    C. The basivertebral veins are seen as high signal structures in MRI images
    D. There are internal and external vertebral venous plexuses
    E. Multiple valves are seen between the segmental veins and vertebral venous plexuses
    F. Epidural venous plexuses are prominent in the cervical vertebra

27. **Vertebral ossification:**
    A. There are three primary centers of ossification
    B. The primary centers appear at eight weeks
    C. The neurocentral joints fuse by seven years
    D. The neural arches unite earlier in the cervical vertebra
    E. The neurocentral joints unite earlier in the lumbar vertebrae

28. **Secondary centers of ossification for vertebra:**
    A. Spinous processes   B. Transverse processes
    C. Mamillary process   D. Upper surface of vertebra
    E. Lower surface of vertebra

29. **Vertebrae:**
    A. Spina bifida is seen in up to 20% of population in the lumbo-sacral level
    B. Disc space and vertebral height are preserved in block vertebra
    C. Dens has two primary centers of ossification
    D. Failure of segmentation is the cause of transitional vertebra
    E. Lumbar rib is due to formation of costal element in the first lumbar vertebra

30. **Scheurmann's disease:**
    A. Majority of adolescent kyphosis is caused by Scheuermann's
    B. At least 3 vertebrae are involved
    C. Disc space not affected
    D. Wedging due to compression fractures
    E. Kyphosis associated with scoliosis in 75%

31. **Craniovertebral junction:**
    A. Up to 2/3rd of dens can be seen above the Chamberlain's line
    B. Extension of dens, more than 5 mm above the McGregor's line is abnormal
    C. A line bisecting the long axis of clivus should pass through the dens
    D. The digastric line should be 1 cm above the atlanto-occipital joints
    E. Bimastoid line touches the upper tip of dens

32. **Cervical vertebra:**
    A. Tubercle in transverse process is not seen in C7
    B. Vertebral veins pass through foramen transversarium of C7
    C. Flexion extension views may show an offset of 3 mm between the posterior cortical margins
    D. Posterior displacement of the spinolaminar line by up to 4 mm is acceptable at the level of axis
    E. The distance between PLL and spinolaminar line should be at least 13 mm

33. **Vertebrae:**
    A. Foramen transversarium is larger on the right side
    B. Cervical rib is seen in 6%
    C. The superior articular facet in cervical vertebrae are oriented anterosuperiorly
    D. The uncinate process is present at birth
    E. In children, the prevertebral space should never be more than 14 mm

34. **Intervertebral disc:**
    A. The annulus fibrosis is remnant of notochord
    B. The internuclear cleft is due to compacted collagen fibres
    C. The internuclear cleft is not seen in 20% of individuals
    D. When seen, the internuclear cleft is seen in all discs
    E. The discs contribute to 5% of vertebral column height

35. **Vertebral curves:**
    A. There are two primary curves and one secondary curves
    B. The lumbar lordosis is exaggerated in females
    C. The physiological thoracic scoliosis is towards the left side
    D. The most prominent point of cervical lordosis is at C6
    E. The most prominent point of thoracic kyphosis is at D7

36. **The following are synovial joints:**
    A. Neurocentral joints
    B. Atlantoaxial joint
    C. Atlanto-occipital joint
    D. Costotransverse joints
    E. Costovertebral joints

37. **Lumbosacral junction:**
    A. The angle of lumbosacral junction is decreased in erect position than supine position
    B. Lumbarisation of first sacral segment is less common than sacralisation of fifth lumbar vertebra
    C. Anterior indentation of thecal sac at lumbosacral level is abnormal
    D. Prominent epidural veins mimics disc at level of L4/5
    E. Lumbosacral disc is convex and smaller than the other lumbar discs

38. **Atlantoaxial subluxation is seen in:**
    A. Morquio's syndrome
    B. Arnold-Chiari malformation
    C. Retropharyngeal abscess
    D. Down's syndrome
    E. Ankylosing spondylitis

39. **Regarding spine:**
    A. Syndesmophytes do not extend beyond level of endplates
    B. 85% of rheumatoid patients have upper cervical spine changes
    C. Diffuse ankylosis of facet joints is produced by juvenile chronic arthritis
    D. Hypervitaminosis A causes flowing ossification
    E. Paraspinal haematoma lasts for 1 month

40. **Disc space narrowing is a feature of:**
    A. Ochronosis
    B. Lymphoma
    C. Histiocytosis
    D. Scheuermann's disease
    E. DISH
    F. Paget's disease

41. **Lumbar vertebra:**
    A. The facet joint lies at the level of vertebral body
    B. Pars interarticularis corresponds to the collar of the Scotty dog
    C. Progressive increase of interpedicular distance is the rule
    D. Thinning of pedicle is normal in the thoracolumbar junction
    E. All facets are in sagittal plane in the lumbar vertebrae

42. **Platyspondyly is seen in:**
    A. Leukemia
    B. Histiocytosis X
    C. Metastatic neuroblastoma
    D. Paget's
    E. Osteoporosis

43. **Disc calcification is seen in:**
    A. Haemochromatosis
    B. Alkaptonuria
    C. Sarcoidosis
    D. DISH
    E. Sequestered disc

44. **The following statements are true:**
    A. Hydatid disease of the spine destroys the intervertebral disc
    B. Calcification in intervertebral disc is a feature of brucellosis
    C. Loss of anterior concavity in body precedes ligament calcification in ankylosing spondylitis
    D. Anterosuperior beaking occurs in achondroplasia
    E. Paravertebral ossification developing in psoriasis is identical to ankylosing spondylitis

45. **Bone marrow:**
    A. High signal postradiation will be seen within two weeks of 5000 rad treatment
    B. Fatty reconversion seen within 6 weeks
    C. Marrow changes in pelvic bones, seen in 8 days after radiation for cervical carcinoma
    D. Metastasis produces low signal in T1 and high in T2, but myeloma is low in both
    E. T2* images are used as screening sequence for spinal metastasis

46. **Following are features of acute metastatic compression fractures as against acute osteoporotic compression fractures:**
    A. Convex posterior body
    B. Hypointense band in T1 and T2
    C. Abnormal signal intensity in pedicles and posterior elements
    D. Epidural mass
    E. Diffuse paraspinal mass
    F. High signal in diffusion sequences

47. **Thoracic vertebra:**
    A. The vertebrae become large caudally
    B. Costotransverse articulations are seen in all thoracic levels
    C. Two facets are seen for costovertebral articulations at all thoracic levels
    D. Superior articular facet faces posterolaterally
    E. Transverse processes become progressively larger towards the lower end

48. **MRI findings of acute osteoporotic compression fractures:**
    A. Hyperintense band in T1 and T2 weighted images
    B. Areas of normal signal intensity
    C. Retropulsed posterior fragment
    D. Multiple compression fractures
    E. Contrast enhancement
    F. Low signal in diffusion sequences

49. **Fluid sign in MRI:**
    A. Indicates benign fracture
    B. More frequent in benign fractures with complete bone marrow changes
    C. Significant association was seen with severity of fracture
    D. Always linear
    E. Indicates osteonecrosis

50. **Craniovertebral ligaments:**
    A. The apical ligament passes from the apex of dens to the margins of foramen magnum
    B. The alar ligaments limit the rotation of skull on atlas
    C. The transverse ligaments are 6 mm thick
    D. The cruciform ligaments pass only superiorly from the transverse ligament
    E. The tectorial membrane is the continuation of the posterior longitudinal ligament cranially

51. **Spinal canal:**
    A. All the cervical vertebrae show a triangular spinal canal
    B. The lower limit of AP diameter of C7 spinal canal is 15 mm
    C. The thoracic dural sac is larger than the cord
    D. The upper lumbar vertebrae show round canals with equal transverse and AP diameters
    E. The perimedullary space is the lowest in the thoracic level

52. **High signal in diffusion weighted images is produced by:**
    A. Membranes
    B. Tight junctions
    C. Fibres
    D. Macromolecules
    E. Organelles

53. **Causes of anterior vertebral beaking:**
    A. Morquio's syndrome   B. Chondrodysplasia punctata
    C. Down's syndrome   D. Acromegaly
    E. Cretinism

54. **Bone marrow:**
    A. In neonates the bone marrow is red
    B. There is a predictable change in bone marrow appearance
    C. In the adolescents, red marrow is seen at epiphyses
    D. The best sequence to show the difference between red and yellow is T2
    E. Yellow marrow is bright in T1 and T2

55. **Spondylolisthesis:**
    A. Degenerative spondylolisthesis is common in L5-S1 level
    B. Isthmic listhesis is common in L4-5 level
    C. Defect in the pars is developmental
    D. Pain is worse in flexion in the isthmic type
    E. Surgical fusion is advisable if more than 50% slippage in isthmic type

56. **Spondylolisthesis:**
    A. The AP diameter of the spinal canal is increased in the spondylolytic type
    B. The lateral recess is stenosed without stenosis of central canal in degenerative type
    C. Pars defect is usually sclerosed
    D. The pedicle has high signal in T1 and T2 weighted images
    E. Facet joints are vertically oriented in degenerative spondylolisthesis

57. **Vacuum sign in the vertebra is seen in:**
    A. Spondylosis
    B. Multiple myeloma
    C. Metastasis
    D. Osteoporosis
    E. Trauma

58. **Vertebrae:**
    A. Intravertebral vacuum cleft is highly suggestive of avascular necrosis
    B. The vacuum cleft is best seen in flexion view
    C. High signal in T1W images in disc is due to calcification
    D. High signal in T2W images in degenerate disc is due to cracks or fissures
    E. High signal can be seen due to fibrosis

59. **The following show normal enhancement in MRI:**
    A. Disc   B. Facetal joint
    C. Pedicle   D. Paraspinal soft tissue
    E. Intrathecal linear

60. **Vertebrae:**
    A. In Modic Type I, there is low signal in both sequences
    B. In Modic II, fatty changes are seen
    C. In Modic III, low signal in T1 and high signal in T2
    D. Schmorl's node enhances on contrast
    E. In limbus vertebra, the disc herniates through the apophysis

61. **Spine:**
    A. Annular bulge is normal in old patients
    B. Annular bulge can be associated with annular tear
    C. In protrusion, the annulus is intact
    D. Axial images are the best for assessing protrusion
    E. Tear of inner annular fibers can be seen in axial images

62. **Spine:**
    A. Protrusion is seen in asymptomatic individuals
    B. Extrusion is asymptomatic
    C. The posterior annular fibers are disrupted in extrusion
    D. Extruded disc usually extends inferiorly but not superiorly
    E. Extruded disc can be located in the lateral recess

63. **Disc disease:**
    A. Sequestered disc is surrounded by epidural fibrosis
    B. Axial images are best for assessing the posterior aspect of disc
    C. Sagittal images are best for assessing lateral recess stenosis
    D. Degenerate discs are hyperintense in T2* images
    E. Degenerate discs are high signal in T2 images

64. **Disc disease:**
    A. Majority of herniated disc are degenerate
    B. Posterolateral herniation will impinge on nerve root
    C. High signal in herniated disc is normal
    D. T1 is best for assessing disk thecal sac interface .
    E. Nerve roots enhance on contrast administration above the level of impingement

65. **Disc disease:**
    A. Double fragment sign indicates that the posterior longitudinal ligament is intact
    B. The sequestered fragment enhances peripherally
    C. High signal is seen in intradural herniated disc
    D. Calcified facetal cyst is in the same location as extruded cyst
    E. Annular tears do not enhance on contrast

66. **Postoperative spine:**
    A. Epidural scar does not enhance on gadolinium administration
    B. Epidural scar occurs only in discectomy surgeries
    C. Epidural scar can occur postfacetectomy
    D. Epidural scar is the end result of epidural haematoma
    E. Gadolinium should be given in postoperative evaluation only if discectomy has been done

67. **Spine MRI:**
    A. A limited MRI scan (STIR and T1 sagittal) is better for assessing low back pain and radiculopathy not responding to conservative management
    B. STIR is more sensitive than T1W images for sclerotic metastasis
    C. Fracture is better seen in STIR than T1
    D. Limited MRI has high sensitivity
    E. Plain X-ray visualization of lytic process requires loss of 80% of bone

68. **Gross increase in marrow iron content is seen in:**
    A. Thalassemia minor
    B. Myelodysplasia
    C. Aplastic anemia
    D. Hemochromatosis
    E. Anemia of chronic disease

69. **Bone marrow changes:**
    A. Marrow reconversion in pregnancy is seen only if there is iron deficiency anemia
    B. Bone marrow signal is more in homogeneous in females than males
    C. Marrow heterogeneity is seen in heavy smokers
    D. Marathon runners have heterogeneous bone marrow in all the bones of the body
    E. Obesity is not a known cause of bone marrow inhomogeneity

70. **Vascular supply to femur:**
    A. The nutrient artery of femur is close to the knee joint
    B. Two-thirds of supply to the head is from lateral epiphyseal arteries
    C. The vascular ring supplying the femoral head is completely within the hip joint capsule
    D. The artery of ligamentum teres is from obturator artery
    E. The retinacular arteries lie within the capsule outside the synovial membrane

71. **Bone marrow changes:**
    A. In anorexia nervosa, the marrow is depleted and shows fatty signals only
    B. Excess fatty replacement is seen in aplastic anemia
    C. In Paget's disease, low signal is seen in T1 and high signal in T2
    D. Transient regional osteoporosis shows low signal in T1, high signal in T2 and STIR
    E. Regional osteoporosis spares the acetabulum

72. **Bone marrow changes:**
    A. Red marrow is isointense in T2* images
    B. Gaucher's disease—high signal in both T1 and T2
    C. Leukemia can produce only diffuse marrow infiltration
    D. Chemical shift imaging can measure the exact amount of fat deposited after chemotherapy
    E. There will be flare up of disease after chemotherapy, but this is not significant

73. **Quantitative T1 relaxation measurement of bone marrow:**
    A. Useful mainly in children
    B. Elevated if more than 350 ms
    C. Elevated in leukemia
    D. Low in rhabdomyosarcoma
    E. Low in metastatic neuroblastoma

74. **The following are causes of spinal stenosis:**
    A. Paget's disease
    B. Spondylolisthesis
    C. DISH
    D. Fluorosis
    E. Achondroplasia

75. **Spinal stenosis:**
    A. More common in the thoracic than cervical region
    B. Cervical canal is stenosed if it measures less than 15 mm
    C. The cervical spinal canal is normally smaller in children
    D. In normal persons, the AP dimension of the spinal canal/AP dimension of vertebral body is less than 1
    E. The dorsal aspect of the canal is compressed more during hyperflexion

76. **The following dimensions are suggestive of lumbar spinal stenosis:**
    A. AP midsagittal diameter in plain film < 15 mm
    B. Transverse diameter (interpedicular distance) < 25 mm
    C. CT area < 1.45 cm^2
    D. CT AP dimension < 15 mm
    E. CT transverse diameter < 10 mm

77. **Anatomy of spinal canal:**
    A. The transverse diameter of lumbar canal increases from L1 to L5
    B. The AP diameter of lumbar canal increases from L1 to L5
    C. L4-5 is the most common segment involved in spinal stenosis
    D. Trefoil shape is normal in L4/5
    E. Spinal claudication reduces on sitting down

78. **Common causes of narrowing of spinal canal:**
    A. Achondroplasia
    B. Ligamentum flavum hypertrophy
    C. Spondylolisthesis
    D. Proximal placement of dorsal root ganglia
    E. Hypertrophied bone graft

79. **Spinal stenosis:**
    A. Lateral recess is stenosed when it is less than 7 mm
    B. The lateral recess is measured at the superior portion of pedicle close to the superior articular facet
    C. Radicular canal is extradural
    D. The intervertebral foramen size decreases from T12-L1 to L4-5
    E. The largest nerve root is through the L5-S1

80. **Spinal stenosis:**
    A. Neurogenic claudication begins after walking for some distance, progressively increases and is relieved by rest
    B. Root pain is due to interference with arterial supply
    C. Motor symptoms appear earlier than sensory symptoms on walking
    D. Posterolateral osteophytes usually arise from the pedicles
    E. In lateral recess stenosis the nerve root is entrapped

81. **Craniovertebral junction:**
    A. The center of gravity of skull passes through the atlanto-occipital joints
    B. The anterior atlanto-occipital membrane has a defect through which the vertebral artery passes through
    C. Rotation of head occurs at the atlanto-occipital joints
    D. The atlanto-occipital joints cannot perform lateral flexion, which is limited by the lateral atlanto-occipital membrane
    E. Tonsillar descent up to 5 mm is normal

82. **Causes of narrowed radicular canal:**
    A. Synovial cyst   B. Hypertrophied articular processes
    C. Disc protrusion   D. Spondylolisthesis
    E. Hypertrophied pedicles

83. **Hips:**
    A. Ultrasound is good in diagnosing hip effusions
    B. Acetabular fractures usually involve the pubis
    C. Early signs of Perthes include widening of the joint space
    D. Pubic symphysis—secondary cartilaginous
    E. Ischium and inferior pubic ramus—synchondroses

84. **Labral tear in hip joint:**
    A. T2 MRI is the most sensitive method
    B. Ganglion cyst is lined by connective tissue cells
    C. Paralabral cysts are associated with congenital hip dysplasia
    D. Labral tear is painless, since there is no neural supply
    E. A paralabral cyst always indicates a labral abnormality

85. **Pelvis:**
    A. The triradiate cartilage fuses 20 years
    B. The center for iliac crest appears at puberty
    C. The anterior inferior iliac spine has a separate ossification center
    D. The pelvic inlet forms an angle of 15 degrees to the horizontal
    E. The pelvic outlet forms an angle of 60 degrees to the horizontal

86. **The following are characteristics of male pelvis:**
    A. Narrower pelvic inlet
    B. Smaller ischial spines
    C. Bigger angle of pubic arch
    D. Prominent sacral promontory
    E. Deeper pelvic cavity

87. **Muscles and their origins:**
    A. Anterior inferior iliac spine—sartorius
    B. Anterior superior iliac spine—straight head of rectus femoris
    C. Piriformis—sacrum
    D. Quadratus femoris—ischial tuberosity
    E. Gemelli superior—ischial spine

88. **Muscles and insertion:**
    A. Piriformis—lesser trochanter
    B. Obturator internus—greater trochanter
    C. Gluteus maximus—greater trochanter
    D. Gluteus minimus—gluteal tuberosity
    E. Obturator externus—lesser trochanter

89. **Structures running through greater sciatic foramen:**
    A. Obturator internus   B. Piriformis
    C. Superior gluteal nerve D. Inferior gluteal artery
    E. Posterior cutaneous nerve of thigh

90. **Ligaments of pelvis:**
    A. The inguinal ligament is a condensation of the external oblique aponeurosis
    B. The sacrotuberous ligament attaches to the posterior inferior iliac spine
    C. Iliolumbar ligament will calcify in old age
    D. The sacrospinous ligament is attached to the posterior inferior iliac spine
    E. Iliolumbar ligament extends from transverse process of L4

91. **Pelvis:**
    A. There are four sacral foramina
    B. The sacral side of the sacroiliac joint is covered by fibrocartilage
    C. The interosseous sacroiliac ligament in the strongest ligament in the body
    D. No movement is possible in the sacroiliac joint
    E. The lumbosacral joint is cartilaginous

92. **Pelvimetry:**
    A. MRI is now the standard modality for pelvimetry
    B. Higher kv is used if standard X-rays are taken
    C. Conjugate diameter less than 10.5 cm indicates cephalopelvic disproportion
    D. Transverse inlet diameter should be more than 12 cm for safe delivery
    E. The minimum bispinous diameter should be 10 cm

93. **Hip joint:**
    A. The articular cartilage completely covers the head of femur
    B. The acetabular cartilage is thickest and strongest inferiorly
    C. The acetabular labrum deepens the articular surface
    D. The transverse acetabular ligament bridges the acetabular notch
    E. The capsule is attached posteriorly to the intertrochanteric crest

94. **Hip joint:**
    A. The ischiofemoral ligament is a thickening of the posterior capsule
    B. The ischiofemoral ligament is attached to the greater trochanter
    C. The pectineus is related anteriorly to the hip joint
    D. Abduction is mainly peformed by gluteus medius and minimus
    E. Extension of hip joint is mainly performed by hamstrings

95. **Femur:**
    A. The neck makes an angle of 135 degrees with the shaft
    B. The neck is anteverted by 8 degrees
    C. In children the neck is anteverted by 50 degrees
    D. The shaft of the femur is angled medially by ten degrees, more in females
    E. The lower end of the shaft is angled backwards on the upper end by 17 degrees

96. **Hip joint:**
    A. The capsule is strongest anteriorly and superiorly
    B. The synovium of hip joint communicates with the psoas bursa through a defect in the fibrous capsule
    C. The ileofemoral ligament is attached to the posterior inferior iliac spine
    D. The articular surface of femoral head is thickest in the center
    E. The pubofemoral ligament is attached only to the pubic ramus superiorly

ANSWERS

1. **A-T, B-T, C-T, D-T, E-F**

   Tuberculosis, lymphoma and aortic aneurysm are the most common causes of anterior scalloping. In tuberculosis, the infection starts in the anterior inferior subchondral region and commonly spreads under the anterior longitudinal ligament causing scalloping of anterior aspect of the vertebra. Aortic aneurysm produces pressure erosion on the portion of the vertebra under the aneurysmal segment. Presence of para-aortic nodes in lymphoma and metastatic cervical carcinoma are other causes.

2. **A-F, B-F, C-T, D-T, E-F**

   There are 33 vertebrae and 31 spinal nerves. The vertebra has three columns. The anterior—ant vertebral body, ant annulus fibrosus, ant long ligament; middle—post body, post ann fibrosus, post long lig; postneural arch. Disruption of PLL without damage to annulus fibrosis or postvertebral body will not cause instability.

3. **A-T, B-T, C-T, D-F, E-T**

   The value of CSF value is close to 0 HU.

4. **A-T, B-T, C-F, D-F, E-F**

   Dorsal root ganglia, meninges and blood vessels enhance.
   Spinal cord, nerve roots and disc do not enhance.

5. **A-T, B-T, C-F, D-F, E-F**

   Red marrow in children will enhance. Blood vessels with rapid flow do not enhance.

6. **A-T, B-F, C-T, D-T, E-T**

   Disc changes are early seen in T2W images.

7. **A-F, B-F, C-T, D-T, E-T**

   2/3rd of trabeculae are vertical and bear the weight, whereas the remaining horizontal trabeculae are horizontal and thin and are only connecting. The superior articular facet faces posteriorly and the inferior articular facet faces anteriorly.

8. **A-F, B-T, C-T, D-F, E-T**

   The discs are thinnest in the upper thoracic region and thicker in the lumbar regions. The discs are thicker anteriorly in the lordotic regions of cervical and lumbar vertebra. The nerve fibres innervate only the peripheral portions of the annulus fibrosus and longitudinal ligaments.

9. **A-F, B-T, C-T, D-T, E-T**
   The supraspinous ligament extends only from C7. It is ligamentum nuchae above this level.

10. **A-T, B-F, C-T, D-T, E-T, F-T**
    The disc is made up of fibrocartilage. The annulus is made up of type I collagen. Nucleus has up to 90% of water.

11. **A-T, B-T, C-T, D-T, E-T**
    Biconcave vertebrae—cause widening of disc space. Osteomalacia, platyspondyly are other causes.

12. **A-F, B-T, C-T, D-T, E-T**
    The cervical canals are oriented anterolaterally and hence oblique views are required for good demonstration. Epidural fat is less in the cervical region, hence the foraminal veins support the nerves. The canal is widest superiorly, where the nerve roots pass through, and are surrounded by foraminal fat, which is maximum in the lumbar region. Transforaminal ligament is occasionally seen, in the lumbar and thoracic region, decreasing the space. The canal narrows with extension, due to sliding of the facets.

13. **A-F, B-F, C-T, D-T, E-F**
    The first seven cervical nerve roots, exit above the level of the corresponding pedicles. All the other nerves exit below the pedicles. C8 nerve root will exit at C7/T1 level.
    Lumbar ganglia are easily identified.

14. **A-F, B-T, C-F, D-T, E-T,**
    Sympathetic fibers are carried along the ventral nerve roots.
    The cervical roots exit horizontally, the thoracic bend downwards and then upwards and the lumbar almost vertically downwards. The lumbar roots exit below the level of intervertebral discs except S1, which exits above.
    Conjoined root is seen in 1%, common at lumbosacral level.

15. **A-T, B-F, C-T, D-T, E-F**
    Ankle—S1, 2. Triceps—C6,7

16. **A-T, B-F, C-T, D-T, E-T**
    Flexion of spine, increases the interspinous distance and also causes cranial migration of cord. Cervical puncture performed in prone or supine position.

17. **A-F, B-F, C-F, D-F, E-T**
    ALL—broadens inferiorly. Attached to bodies but not to discs. Three layers. The deepest joins adjacent vertebra, middle 2-3 vertebra and superficial 4-5 vertebra.

PLL—tapers inferiorly. Continues superiorly as tectal membrane. Attached to disc. Separated from body by basivertebral vein and venous plexus.

18. **A-T, B-T, C-T, D-F, E-T**
The epidural fat is seen anteriorly within the V of ligamentum flavum. Ligamentum flavum is elastic.

19. **A-T, B-F, C-F, D-T, E-F**
Facet joints are synovial joints with a capsule, hyaline cartilage and synovial membrane. The inferior articular process is situated posteriorly to the superior articular process. The nerves are from the same level and above the level. Menisci are seen only in cervical joints. Cervical joints are 45 degrees, thoracic 60 degrees, lumbar 45 degrees and lumbosacral joint—coronal.

20. **A-T, B-F, C-T, D-T, E-T**
OPLL seen in 6th decade. Starts from C4/5 or C3/4 and extends to thoracic spine. Disc can enhance in delayed scan.

21. **A-F, B-F, C-F, D-T, E-T**
Flexor muscles are supplied by anterior primary rami and extensors by posterior primary rami. Sternocleidomastoid and rectus abdominis are the major flexors in neck and abdomen. The oblique muscles of abdomen are the major rotators.

22. **A-F, B-T, C-F, D-T, E-T**
Uncovertebral joints (Luschka's joints) in cervical region are synovial. Intervertebral joints are fibrous. Cervical spine shows flexion, extension, rotation and lateral flexion. The flexion is limited by tension in the extensor muscles. Rotation occurs mainly in the thoracic spine. Other movements are not possible. Flexion and extension occurs in the lumbar spine, but rotation is limited.

23. **A-T, B-T, C-T, D-T, E-T**
Multiple sclerosis, trauma, syringomyelia after collapse, cord infarction, radiation, syphilis, subacute combined degeneration are other causes.

24. **A-T, B-T, C-T, D-T, E-F**
Degenerative disease, vertebral fusion, unilateral bar with scoliosis are other causes, neurofibroma, dermoids, hypoplastic pedicles, dural ectasia (Marfan's, Ehlers-Danlos), hydatid, ligamental fibroma, neuropathies are other causes.

25. **A-T, B-T, C-T, D-T, E-T**
Neural elements constitute 25% of foramen.

26. **A-F, B-F, C-T, D-T, E-F, F-T**

    Segmental supply is from ascending pharyngeal, occipital, thyrocervical and costocervical trunk to cervical and branches from aorta to dorsolumbar vertebrae. The lateral sacral artery supplies the sacrum.

    Although the segmental vertebral arteries supply the corresponding side of the vertebral, the right intercostal arteries also supply the anterior aspect of the left side of vertebra also. Basivertebral veins drain the vertebra. They are less prominent in cervical vertebrae. Two channels are seen in lumbar and three in thoracic level. They are of high signal due to slow flow and perivenous fat. They create a notch in the posterior vertebral body. There are anterior and posterior epidural venous plexus inside the spinal canal. These are very prominent in cervical level and enhance on contrast. These drain into the external vertebral venous plexus which drains into segmental veins. There are no valves in these veins.

27. **A-T, B-T, C-T, D-F, E-F**

    There is one center for the centrum and two for the neural arches. The neurocentral joints join earlier in the cervical vertebrae and the neural arches join earlier in the lumbar level.

28. **A-T, B-T, C-T, D-T, E-T**

    The centers appear at puberty and fuse in early 20s. Those for vertebral body fuse by 30 years.

29. **A-T, B-F, C-T, D-T, E-T**

    Spina bifida is due to failure of fusion of neural arches, and is seen in up to 20% of population, and less than 4 mm. Block vertebra and transitional vertebra are due to failure of segmentation. In block vertebra, the disc space is narrowed but the overall height is preserved. Lumbar and cervical rib are due to development of costal elements in these levels.

30. **A-F, B-T, C-F, D-F, E-T**

    Normal kyphosis in adolescents is 20-40%. Majority are postural. In Scheuermann's kyphosis, 3 or more consecutive vertebrae are wedge due to remodelling by at least 5 degrees. Decreased disc height, increased AP dimension, irregular end plates and Schmorl's nodes are seen.

31. **A-F, B-F, C-T, D-T, E-T**

    Chamberlain's line—hard palate to posterior lip of foramen magnum—1/3rd or 5 mm of dens can be above this line. McGregor's line—hard palate to inferior surface of occipital bone—7 mm of dens can be above this. Basion is the postero-inferior margin of clivus and opisthion is the anterior limit of occipital bone.

32. **A-T, B-T, C-T, D-F, E-T**
C7 foramen is small or absent, and may transmit only vertebral veins.
Due to long spinous process, the spinolaminar line may be displaced up to 2 mm at level of axis.
Axis is the strongest cervical vertebra. Atlas has no body and only lateral masses are seen. Vertebral artery and suboccipital nerve pass through the arcuate foramen which is due to calcification of atlanto-occipital membrane. The odontoid has more compact bone than the body, making it more darker in MRI.

33. **A-F, B-T, C-T, D-F, E-T**
Foramen transversarium is larger on left side. Sup facet is anterosuperiorly placed and inf facet is placed posteroinferiorly. The uncinate process is not present at birth. In adults, prevertebral space can be up to 22 mm.

34. **A-F, B-T, C-F, D-T, E-F**
The nucleus pulposus is the notochord remnant. The internuclear cleft is compacted collagen fibres due to invagination of inner lamella and is seen after 30 yr, not seen in 6% and seen in all discs when seen. The discs contribute to 20% of vertebral height.

35. **A-F, B-T, C-F, D-F, E-T**
The thoracic and pelvic kyphosis are primary, present at birth. The lumbar and cervical lordosis are secondary.
Cervical—from atlas to D2. prominent at C4.
Thoracic—from D2-D12. Most prominent at D7. Physiological scoliosis to the right side.
Lumbar—from L1-L5. More in females. Prominent at L3.
Pelvic—up to coccyx.

36. **A-T, B-T, C-T, D-T, E-T**

37. **A-F, B-T, C-T, D-T, E-T**
In supine position the angle is 25-55 degrees and in erect it increases by 8-12 degrees.
Lumbosacral disc is smaller (5 mm), convex and there is large amount of epidural fat.

38. **A-T, B-F, C-T, D-T, E-T**
Atlantoaxial subluxation—atlantodental space > 5 mm children, > 3 mm adults.

Congenital—Congenital absence/hypoplasia of dens, Down's, Morquio's, spondyloepiphyseal dysplasia, trauma
Inflammatory—RA, JRA, ank spondylitis, psoriasis,
Infection—Retropharyngeal abscess (Grisel's syndrome).

39. **A-T, B-T, C-F, D-T, E-T**
AS and JRA are the common causes of diffuse ankylosis of facet joints. DISH, degeneration, hypertrophic osteoarthropathy, fluorosis, retinoid toxicity also cause flowing ossification.

40. **A-T, B-T, C-F, D-T, E-F, F-T**
Tuberculosis, pyogenic infections are the most common causes. Fluorosis, myelofibrosis, mastocytosis, renal osteodystrophy, neuropathic, RA, axial osteomalacia are other causes.

41. **A-F, B-T, C-T, D-T, E-F**
The facet joint is in the sagittal plane and is seen at the level of the intervertebral disc. The sagittal plane prevents lateral rotation. In the lumbosacral level, the facets are oriented coronal plane, with inferior articular facet oriented anteriorly. Thinning of pedicle is seen in 7% in thoracolumbar junction.

42. **A-T, B-T, C-T, D-F, E-T**
Platyspondyly is flattening of the vertebral bodies. It is commonly seen in metastasis. Involvement of multiple vertebra is characteristic of spondyloepiphyseal dysplasia. It is also seen in Morquio's disease.

43. **A-T, B-T, C-F, D-T, E-T**
Spondylosis, CPDD (calcium pyrophosphate dihydrate deposition disease) idiopathic, ankylosing spondylitis, gout, juvenile chronic arthritis, spinal fusion are other causes.

44. **A-F, B-F, C-T, D-F, E-F**
Hydatid disease is not very common in the spine. It is seen as a lytic lesion, which expands the cortex. Usually, the intervertebral discs are not involved. In achondroplasia, there is anteroinferior beaking. In Morquio's, there is middle beaking. In AS, annulus fibrosis is ossified. In psoriasis, paravertebral ossification, separated from vertebral body and disc.

45. **A-T, B-F, C-T, D-F, E-F**
Metastasis and myeloma produce the same signal changes and hence cannot be reliably differentiated in T1 and T2. STIR images are used as the screening sequence, since any pathological lesion of significance will be bright in this sequence.

46. **A-T, B-T, C-T, D-T, E-F, F-T**

Differentiating a metastatic compression fracture and an osteoporotic compression fracture in an elderly patient is extremely difficult. Some of the features in favour of a metastasis are, 1. a convex posterior aspect of vertebral body, 2. abnormal signal intensity in pedicles and posterior elements, 3. encasing epidural mass, 4. focal paraspinal mass, 5. involvement of adjacent vertebra, and 6. completely changed bone marrow signal (metastatis frequently collapses only after the entire bone has been involved). The first two can also be seen in osteoporotic collapse. Diffuse paraspinal mass is nonspecific. Focal paraspinal mass is frequent in metastasis. Hypointense band is a feature of osteoporosis. Diffusion imaging is the recent modality used for differentiating. Metastasis appears as high signal and osteoporotic fractures are low signal. Although some osteoporotic fractures may be high signal, progressively increasing the diffusion gradient will ultimately result in low signal in osteoporosis, but always high in tumour.

47. **A-T, B-F, C-F, D-T, E-F**

The first three vertebrae decrease in caliber, but from this level, there is progressive increase in size. Transverse processes become progressively smaller. Costotransverse articulations are seen from D1-10. Costo vertebral articulations have two facets from D2-10. Only single facet is seen in the other levels. Superior articular facet faces posterolaterally and inf facet anteromedially.

48. **A-F, B-T, C-T, D-T, E-F, F-T**

Features of a benign osteoporotic compression fracture in an MRI are: 1. hypointense band in T1 and T2W images, 2. Sparing of normal bone marrow signal (may not be spared if reactive changes extend all around), 3. Retropulsion of posterior fragment, 4. multiple compression fractures. The signal intensity and contrast enhancement features are not very helpful in differentiating. Metastasis is usually hypo to iso in T1 and hyper or heterogeneous in T2 and show heterogeneous intense enhancement, findings which may be frequently seen in osteoporotic fractures also. Diffusion images demonstrate low signal in osteoporotic compression. Occasionally, they may be iso or hyperintense, but increasing the diffusion gradient will make the lesion hypointense, unlike metastasis which is unaltered.

49. **A-T, B-T, C-T, D-F, E-T**

Fluid sign is the presence of a linear or triangular fluid signal adjacent to end plate, in a STIR image, seen specifically in benign fractures (only occasionally in metastatic). In a patient with osteoporosis, minor trauma will result in compression fracture. This is associated with fracture of the end plate, which will result in osteonecrosis due to compression of trabeculae. The fluid sign is caused by collection of fluid in the region of osteonecrosis.

50. **A-F, B-T, C-T, D-F, E-T**
Apical ligament—from apex of dens to anterior midpoint of foramen magnum. Alar ligament—from apex of dens to occipital condyles. Transverse ligament—between the tubercles in anterior margin of atlas. Cruciform ligament—from transverse ligament, superiorly to basiocciput and inferiorly to body of axis. Atlanto-occipital membranes—from upper borders of anterior and posterior arches of atlas to respective border of foramen magnum.

51. **A-F, B-F, C-T, D-T, E-T**
The cervical vertebrae are triangular except the atlas which is round. The thoracic and upper lumbar are also round. The lower lumbar are triangular. The lower limit of atlas is 16 mm, axis 15 mm and others 12 mm. In dorsolumbar it is 15 mm. The perimedullary space is between the cord and bony canal and is maximum of 8 mm in cervical and 3 mm in thoracic spine.

52. **A-T, B-T, C-T, D-T, E-T**
Restricted fluid also produces high signal in diffusion weighted images.

53. **A-T, B-F, C-T, D-F, E-T**
Achondroplasia, Hurler's syndrome, pseudoachondroplasia are other causes.

54. **A-T, B-F, C-T, D-F, E-T**
Red marrow is hypo in T1, hyper in T2, Yellow marrow is hyper in T1 and severe signal in T2. Hence T1 is best for differentiating. The marrow conversion is not predictable.

55. **A-F, B-F, C-T, D-F, E-T**
Degenerative listhesis is common in L4-5 level and isthmic (spondylolytic) L5-S1 level.
Pain in isthmic type is worse in hyperextension.

56. **A-T, B-F, C-T, D-T, E-T**
In spondylolytic type, the AP diameter of canal is increased, but there may be lateral recess stenosis with nerve compression. In degenerative type, the canal diameter is decreased. Facet joints are vertically oriented with erosion of superior medial aspect of inferior facet.

57. **A-T, B-F, C-F, D-T, E-T**
Vacuum sign in the disc is seen due to degenerative disease. Can be seen inside vertebrae due to Schmorl's node/cyse/osteonecrosis. Vacuum cleft within vertebra is an indicator of benign nature of the compression. Apophyseal joints—degenerative, synovial cyst.

58. **A-T, B-F, C-T, D-T, E-T**
Vacuum cleft is best seen in extension. This is a linear lucency within collapsed body. This is not seen in infection/neoplasm.

59. **A-T, B-T, C-F, D-F, E-T**
The disc can enhance parallel to the endplate.

60. **A-F, B-T, C-F, D-T, E-T**
Modic changes
I—Hypo, hyper—vascular
II—hyper, hyper—fat
III—hypo, hypo—sclerosis

61. **A-T, B-T, C-F, D-T, E-F**
In annular bulge there is diffuse bulging due to loosening of annular fibers. In protrusion, the inner annulus fibers are torn, with intact outer fibers. This tear is difficult to visualise in imaging.

62. **A-T, B-F, C-T, D-F, E-T**
Protrusion is usually seen in asymptomatic individuals but extrusion is usually symptomatic. In extrusion the annulus fibrosis is disrupted with herniation of nucleus pulposus, and can extend either superiorly or inferiorly or laterally.

63. **A-T, B-F, C-F, D-T, E-F**
Sagittal images are best for assessing the posterior aspect of disc, outer annulus fibers and interface with thecal sac. Axial images are best for assessing lateral recess and nerve root.
Normally, hydrated discs are low signal in T1 and high signal in T2. In degeneration, low signal in both sequences due to dehydration. High signal will be seen in T2* images.

64. **A-T, B-T, C-F, D-F, E-T**
High signal in herniated disc denotes either inflammation or increased water in the disc.
T2 is best for assessing the disk thecal sac interface. Nerve roots above the level of impingement are enlarged and enhance on contrast.

65. **A-F, B-T, C-T, D-F, E-T**
Double fragment sign indicates the presence of a hypointense band between the parent disk and extruded fragment, indicating that

the posterior longitudinal ligament has been breached. Annular tears and sequestered fragment can enhance due to peripheral vascular ingrowth. Calcified facetal joint cysts are usually situated posterolateral to thecal sac, discs—anterolateral.

66. **A-F, B-F, C-T, D-T, E-F**

Epidural scars are the end result of epidural haematoma during spinal surgeries. It commonly occurs in discectomy, but it can also be seen in laminectomy, facetectomy and any procedure which results in exploration of posterior annulus fibrosis which causes epidural bleed. So contrast should be administered in any back pain after any back surgery. Enhancement occurs due to rich capillary network in the epidural scar. No enhancement will be seen in recurrent DISC, which is avascular.

67. **A-F, B-F, C-F, D-T, E-T**

Limited MRI (STIR and T1) is a good examination and is preferable to standard lumbar spine X-rays, which have high radiation and cannot find the discal disease. It is useful in low backache; but if there is radiculopathy; the complete MRI sequences should be performed. This does not require radiologist supervision and is highly sensitive for finding any abnormality in bone, which might require detailed examination later. T1 is better for fractures and sclerotic metastasis. Fracture edema is better seen in STIR images.

68. **A-F, B-T, C-T, D-T, E-F**

Thalassemia minor, sickle cell anemia and anemia of chronic disease cause only minor increase in iron content. Thalassemia major is another major cause of gross increase in iron content.

69. **A-F, B-T, C-T, D-F, E-F**

Marrow reconversion is a term used for the conversion of normal fatty marrow in adults, to red marrow. This is more common in females, due to latent iron deficiency state seen due to menstruation. It is seen in pregnancy due to increased erythropoietin volume and also due to iron deficiency anemia. Obesity is a well-known cause. Marathon runners have heterogeneous signal, but there is sparing of distal femur and proximal tibia.

70. **A-F, B-T, C-F, D-T, E-F**

The nutrient artery of femur is in the proximal aspect, away from the knee joint. In tibia and fibula they are close to the ankle joint. Majority of blood supply to femur comes from the lateral epiphyseal branches, which run on the posterosuperior surface of the head, and interrupted in fracture neck, producing avascular necrosis. The vascular ring is within capsule anteriorly and just outside it in the posterior aspect. Artery of ligamentum teres is branch of obturator and medial circumflex femoral A. The retinacular branches are within the capsule beneath the synovial membrane. The femur has one or two nutrient arteries.

71. **A-F, B-T, C-F, D-T, E-T**
There are two patterns in anorexia nervosa. In the common pattern, there is fatty replacement of the bone marrow. In serous atrophy type, there is increased hyaluronic acid, hence, there is low signal in T1 and high in T2. In Paget's disease, low signal is seen in T1 and T2, high signal in only STIR.

72. **A-T, B-F, C-F, D-T, E-T**
Red marrow is hypo in T1, intermediately bright in T2, iso in T2*, bright in STIR. Gaucher's is characterized by deposition of glucocerebroside and hence is low in T1 and T2. Leukemia generally produces diffuse marrow infiltration, but in acute myelogenous leukemia, focal infiltration can be seen. After chemotherapy, the bone marrow initially undergoes hypoplasia, followed by reconversion and then fibrosis. After chemotherapy, the edema in the bone marrow can increase and this may be mistaken for progression of lesion.

73. **A-T, B-F, C-T, D-F, E-F**
In children, bone marrow is mainly red. Any pathological lesion is also of similar signal to bone marrow, i.e. low signal in T1 and high signal in T2. Hence, quantitative measurements of bone marrow T1 relaxation time may be of help. The normal time is 350-650 ms. It is abnormal, if more than 750 ms. It is elevated in leukemia, metastasis and rhabdomyosarcoma.

74. **A-T, B-T, C-T, D-T, E-T**
Degenerative disease is the most common cause of spinal stenosis. Other causes include congenital, developmental, spondylolisthesis, acromegaly, postsurgical, trauma, fibrous dysplasia, severe kyphosis, scoliosis and ankylosing spondylosis.

75. **A-F, B-F, C-F, D-F, E-F**
Spinal stenosis is more in cervical region than in thoracic region. Normal cervical canal measures more than 13 mm. Less than 10 mm is spinal stenosis. The AP diameter of spinal canal/AP diameter of vertebral body is normally more than 1 in stenosis it is less than 0.8. The canal is larger in normal children than adults. The dorsal aspect of the canal is compressed more during hyperextension.

76. **A-T, B-F, C-T, D-F, E-F**
    The AP midsagittal diameter is measured in plain film between the posterior surface of vertebral body to the base of superior articular facet. Normal is more than 15 mm. Some use 12 mm as normal measurement. 10-12 mm as relative stenosis and < 10 mm as absolute stenosis. Transverse interpediculate distance less than 20 mm is stenotic.
    CT, AP < 11.5 mm, transverse < 16 mm and area < 1,45 cm^2 are features of stenosis.

77. **A-T, B-F, C-T, D-T, E-T**
    The AP diameter of the lumbar canal decreases from L1 to L5. The most common segment involved are L4-5 and L5-S1. Spinal claudication is absent at rest, back pain and walking, with relief on sitting or crouching. The normal lumbar canal is triangular with smooth angles.

78. **A-T, B-T, C-F, D-F, E-T**
    Osteophytes, postoperative changes are other causes of spinal canal narrowing. Spondylolisthesis and proximal placement of dorsal root ganglia are causes of narrowing of intervertebral foramen along with disc, osteophytes, tumours, infection, synovial cysts, and fibrosis.

79. **A-F, B-T, C-T, D-F, E-T**
    Lateral recess is bounded anteriorly by posterior surface of vertebral body and disc, laterally by medial margin of pedicle and posteriorly by superior facet. Normally, it is more than 5 mm. 3-5 mm is highly suggestive of stenosis and less than 3 mm is definitive stenosis. Radicular canal is between the central part of spinal canal and intervertebral foramen. The intervertebral foramen increases from T12 to L5. The L5/S1 has the smallest foramen and has the largest nerve root.

80. **A-F, B-T, C-F, D-F, E-F**
    Neurogenic claudication begins rapidly on walking, progressively increases with appearance of sensory symptoms followed by motor symptoms, not relieved by rest, but relieved by stooping or crouching. Root pain can also be due to venous congestion or interference with CSF drainage. Anterior osteophytes arise from endplates, lateral from pedicles and posterolateral from apophyseal joints. In lateral recess stenosis the nerve is not entrapped but medially displaced.

81. **A-F, B-F, C-F, D-F, E-T**
    Center of gravity passes anterior to level of atlanto-occipital joints. Rotation of head occurs at atlantoaxial joints. Flexion, extension

and lateral flexion occurs at atlanto-occipital joints. The defect is seen in the posterior atlanto-occipital membrane, transmitting, vertebral artery and upper cervical nerve.

82. A-F, B-T, C-T, D-T, E-T

83. A-T, B-T, C-T, D-T, E-T
Pubic symphysis has two articular surfaces coated by hyaline cartilage, with intervening fibrocartilaginous disc.

84. A-F, B-T, C-T, D-F, E-T
MR arthrography is the most sensitive method, with 91% accuracy. Pathologically, there are two types of paralabral cysts, the ganglion cysts and synovial cysts. These cannot be differentiated radiologically. They are commonly seen with osteoarthritis, trauma and congenital hip dysplasia. Labrum is supplied by nerves and hence a labral tear is very painful and produces clicks.

85. A-T, B-T, C-T, D-F, E-F
The pelvic inlet is 50-60 degrees to horizontal and outlet is 15 degrees. The triradiate cartilage appears at puberty and fuses at 20 years. The center for iliac crest and ischial tuberosity also appears at pubery and fuses by 20 years.

86. A-T, B-F, C-F, D-T, E-T
Pelvic inlet—narrower; pelvic cavity—deeper; sacrum—longer; sacral alae—narrower than body of sacrum; sacral promontory—prominent; ischial spines—prominent; pubic arch—smaller; muscle attachments—prominent.

87. A-F, B-F, C-T, D-T, E-T
Anterior superior iliac spine—sartorius. Anterior inferior iliac spine—straight head of rectus femoris. Gemelli superior from ischial spine and G inferior from ischial tuberosity.

88. A-F, B-T, C-F, D-F, E-F
Piriformis—upper border of greater trochanter; obturator internus—medial greater trochanter; obturator externus—trochanteric fossa in medial greater trochanter
Gluteus maximus—gluteal tuberosity:
Gluteus minimus and medius—anterior and lateral aspects of greater trochanter.

89. A-F, B-T, C-T, D-T, E-T
Obturator internus runs through lesser sciatic foramen.
Greater sciatic foramen—superior gluteal nerve and vessels inferior gluteal nerve and vessels, sciatic nerve, postcutaneous nerve of thigh, piriformis.
Lesser sciatic notch—obturator internus muscle
Both—pudendal nerve and vessels.

90. **A-T, B-T, C-T, D-F, E-F**

    The sacrotuberous ligament—from ischial tuberosity to sacrum, coccyx, posterior inferior iliac spine—Sacrospinous ligament—ischial spine to sacrum and coccyx. Iliolumbar ligament—transverse process of L5 to iliac crest.

91. **A-F, B-T, C-T, D-F, E-T**

    There are four pairs of dorsal foramina and four pairs of ventral foramina, through which the dorsal and ventral rami emerge. The sacral side of sacroiliac joint is covered by fibrocartilage and the iliac side is covered by hyaline cartilage. Mild rotatory movements are possible in the joint, which is increased during pregnancy.

92. **A-T, B-T, C-T, D-F, E-T**

    High kv reduces radiation. Conjugate diameter >10.5 cm, transverse inlet diameter >11 and bispinous diameter >10 cm are essential for safe vaginal delivery.

93. **A-F, B-F, C-T, D-T, E-F**

    The articular cartilage is absent in the center, where the ligamentum teres is attached. The acetabular cartilage is thickest and broadest superiorly. The capsule is attached anteriorly to the intertrochanteric line and posteriorly 10 mm above the intertrochanteric crest.

94. **A-T, B-T, C-T, D-T, E-T**

    Flexion—iliopsoas; Extension—hamstrings; Abduction—G. minimus and medius; Adduction—Adductors and gracilis; Medial rotation—anterior fibers of G minimus and medius; Lateral rotation—Quadratus.

95. **A-T, B-T, C-T, D-T, E-T**

    The anteversion is 50 in infants, 30 at 2 years, 25 at 3 years. Females have a valgus of 14 degrees, more than males.

96. **A-T, B-T, C-F, D-T, E-F**

    The ileofemoral ligament is attached to the anterior inferior iliac spine and intertrochanteric line. The pubofemoral ligament attaches above to the ileopectineal line, superior pubic ramus and obturator membrane and down to femoral neck.

9 Soft Tissue and Foot

1. **Soft tissue calcification is seen in:**
   A. Cushing's
   B. Tuberous sclerosis
   C. Lead poisoning
   D. Alkaptonuria
   E. Milk alkali syndrome

2. **Common causes of soft tissue ossification:**
   A. Burns
   B. Melorheostosis
   C. Surgical scar
   D. Guinea worm
   E. Varicose veins

3. **Myositis ossificans traumatica:**
   A. The lesion is in the skeletal muscle
   B. Spares the lateral side of the elbow
   C. Development depends on the severity of the injury
   D. The osteoblasts are formed from damaged periosteum
   E. The most common joint involved is the hand

4. **Myositis ossificans:**
   A. A shell of ossification is seen as frequent as homogeneous ossification
   B. Regression is more common in younger patients
   C. Mature bone is deposited within 6-8 weeks
   D. There is always a clear zone between the periphery of the lesion and the underlying bone
   E. The maturation of the lesion progresses from center to periphery

5. **Parosteal lesions:**
   A. In parosteal osteosarcoma there is a complete lucency between the lesion and the cortex of underlying bone
   B. Periphery is less dense in parosteal osteosarcoma
   C. Periosteal osteosarcoma is denser from periphery
   D. Juxtacortical chondroma produces excavation
   E. Cortical thickening is seen in periosteal osteosarcoma

6. **Bursitis:**
   A. Housemaids knee—suprapatellar bursitis
   B. Clergymans knee—prepatellar bursitis
   C. Miners elbow—olecranon bursitis
   D. Weavers bottom—sartorius bursitis
   E. Footballers hip—greater trochanter

7. **Ligmental calcification:**
   A. Calcification of lateral collateral ligament of knee is Pellegrini-Stieda disease
   B. Calcification of stylohyoid ligament produces dysphagia
   C. Eagle syndrome is calcification of patellar tendon
   D. Achilles tendon commonly calcifies at the site of insertion into calcaneus
   E. DISH involves stylohyoid ligament

8. **Florid reactive periostitis:**
   A. Florid reactive periostitis typically affects the metacarpals
   B. Soft tissue mass is seen in florid reactive periostitis
   C. Cortical destruction is seen
   D. In bizarre parosteal osteochondromatous proliferation there is no pain
   E. Stalk is occasionally seen

9. **Parasites causing calcification:**
   A. *Dracunculus medinensis*
   B. *Paragonimus westermani*
   C. *Trichcuris trichiura*
   D. *Ascaris lumbricoides*
   E. *Armillifer armillates*
   F. *Echinococcus granulosus*

10. **Tumoral calcinosis:**
    A. Secondary to tumours such as osteosarcoma
    B. Common in smaller joints especially around wrist and ankle
    C. Severe pain is produced due to joint restriction
    D. Fluid levels indicate that the disease is active
    E. The majority of affected people have inborn error of phosphate metabolism

11. **Tumoral calcinosis:**
    A. The serum calcium and phosphorus are elevated
    B. The ESR is elevated
    C. It is autosomal recessive
    D. Easy to differentiate from renal osteodystrophy
    E. Antacids are treatment of choice

12. **Parasitic calcification:**
    A. Cysticercosis is not seen in vegetarians
    B. The calcification in cysticercosis is oval and is perpendicular to the direction of muscle fibres
    C. Loa loa calcification is best seen in the hands and feet
    D. Armiller calcification is crescentic and is seen mainly in the limbs
    E. Guinea worm infestation is caused by male worms

13. **Myositis ossificans progressiva:**
    A. Autosomal recessive disease
    B. The primary process is centered in the muscles
    C. Dysplasia of first metatarsal is seen in 75% of cases
    D. Dysplastic changes in the cervical vertebra precede the soft tissue changes
    E. The patients die of respiratory compromise

14. **Myositis ossificans progressiva:**
    A. Elevated alkaline phosphatase
    B. The disease progresses from caudal to cranial
    C. Torticollis is the most frequent symptom
    D. Injections precipitate an acute attack
    E. The most rapid progression happens in the second decade

15. **Associations of myositis ossificans progressiva:**
    A. Conductive deafness
    B. Premature baldness
    C. Hypogonadism
    D. Mental retardation
    E. Leukemia

16. **Causes of calcinosis circumscripta:**
    A. Varicose veins—calf
    B. Hypervitaminosis A
    C. Hypervitaminosis D
    D. Scleroderma
    E. Dermatomyositis

17. **Metastatic calcification is seen in the following locations:**
    A. Gastric mucosa
    B. Heart
    C. Vessels
    D. Bronchial wall
    E. Kidney

18. **Musculoskeletal ultrasound:**
    A. Baker's cyst arises from the lateral head of gastrocnemius
    B. Neurofibromas are seen as cystic lesions with acoustic enhancement
    C. Doppler is better than contrast-enhanced MRI for evaluation of soft tissue masses
    D. MRI of soft tissue masses can be done either before or after biopsy
    E. Follow-up studies for soft tissue masses should always be the same modality

19. **Musculoskeletal ultrasound has the following uses:**
    A. Achilles tendinosis
    B. Supraspinatus tear
    C. Patellar tendinosis
    D. Carpal tunnel syndrome
    E. Tennis elbow
    F. Guidance for steroid injection for tendonitis

20. **Musculoskeletal ultrasound:**
    A. Abnormal striation in muscle is suggestive of muscle tear
    B. Ultrasound can detect a metal fragment as small as 0.3 cm
    C. Ultrasound can detect a wooden FB, as small as 0.7 mm
    D. Ultrasound can detect glass FB as small as 2 mm
    E. Ultrasound can detect plastic FB larger than 2 mm

21. **Causes of carpal tunnel syndrome:**
    A. Renal failure
    B. Rheumatoid arthritis
    C. Gout
    D. Amyloidosis
    E. SLE

22. **Causes of metastatic calcification:**
    A. Leukemia
    B. Myeloma
    C. Bony metastasis
    D. Sarcoidosis
    E. Lung cancer

23. **Vascular calcification is seen in:**
    A. Hyperparathyroidism
    B. Raynaud's syndrome
    C. Mönckeberg's disease
    D. Ehlers-Danlos syndrome
    E. Diabetes

24. The following disorders produce soft tissue calcification without hypercalcemia:
    A. Sarcoidosis
    B. Pseudohypoparathyroidism
    C. Hypoparathyroidism
    D. Renal osteodystrophy
    E. Paget's disease

25. Causes of high signal intensity in muscles in MRI:
    A. Diabetic infarction
    B. Hypokalemia
    C. Alcohol intoxication
    D. Lymphoma
    E. Denervation

26. Diabetic muscular infarction:
    A. Bilateral
    B. Mass palpable
    C. It is due to vascular occlusion
    D. Recurrent
    E. Coexistent diabetic retinopathy and nephropathy seen

27. Diabetic muscular infarction:
    A. Muscle is atrophic
    B. The calf muscles are most common affected group
    C. Isointense in T1
    D. Hyperintense in T1, due to haemorrhage
    E. Contrast enhancement not seen

28. Sports injuries and origin of injury:
    A. Tennis leg—plantaris tendon
    B. Tennis elbow—common extensor origin
    C. Golfers elbow—lateral epicondyle
    D. Runners knee—patella
    E. Shin splints—tibialis posterior

29. Musculoskeletal ultrasound:
    A. At least 5 ml of fluid should be present in pediatric hip to diagnose effusion
    B. Tendons are seen as hyperechoic structures
    C. Duchenne's muscular dystrophy, the muscle becomes more echogenic
    D. Spinal canal stenosis can be diagnosed in adults
    E. Depth of acetabulum can be assessed in children

30. **Features of tennis leg:**
    A. Fluid between aponeurosis of medial head of gastrocnemius and soleus
    B. Ruptured soleus
    C. Ruptured plantaris
    D. Deep venous thrombosis
    E. Rupture of gastrocnemius occurs in midportion

31. **Muscle hernias:**
    A. Tibialis anterior is the most common muscle affected
    B. The swelling is prominent after exertion
    C. The fascial defect is usually closed by surgery to treat muscle hernias
    D. Herniated muscle is more echogenic than the normal adjacent muscle
    E. Spoke-like appearance is seen in ultrasound

32. **Causes of heel pain syndrome:**
    A. Stress fracture of calcaneum
    B. Achilles tendonitis
    C. Tarsal tunnel syndrome
    D. Ankylosing spondylitis
    E. Median calcaneal neuritis

33. **Common causes of forefoot pain:**
    A. Freiberg's infraction
    B. Sesamoiditis
    C. Plantar fasciitis
    D. Morton's neuroma
    E. Neuropathic arthropathy

34. **Causes of forefoot pain:**
    A. Ganglia
    B. Calluses
    C. Septic arthritis
    D. Rheumatoid arthritis
    E. Osteoarthritis

35. **Plantar fasciitis:**
    A. Pain is characteristic in the posteromedial aspect of calcaneum
    B. In acute stage the pain is seen at the origin of plantar fascia
    C. Pain exacerbated by plantar flexion of feet
    D. Pain severe in morning
    E. High frequency ultrasound is used to relieve pain

36. **Plantar fasciitis:**
    A. Plantar calcaneal spur is pathognomonic
    B. Heel pad is thickened
    C. Bone scan is normal
    D. Normal plantar fascia measures up to 6 mm
    E. Thickening is focal nodular

37. **Freiberg's infraction:**
    A. Common in women
    B. Seen in adolescent age group
    C. Fifth metatarsal head affected
    D. High heels predisposes
    E. Low signal in T2 weighted image in earliest stage

38. **Talar avascular necrosis:**
    A. Seen in 50% of talar dislocation
    B. The talus is supplied by branch of anterior tibial artery
    C. Diffuse hyperintensity involving whole talus is seen in T2W images
    D. The tarsal canal artery enters through the lateral aspect of tarsal canal
    E. Focal areas of necrosis is seen within the high signal in talus

39. **Tarsal tunnel syndrome:**
    A. Affects anterior tibial nerve
    B. Compression is between flexor digitorum longus and flexor hallucis longus
    C. Seen posterior and inferior to lateral malleolus
    D. Post-traumatic fibrosis is a recognised cause
    E. Entrapment symptoms due to flexor retinaculum

40. **Anatomy of leg:**
    A. The peroneal nerve winds around the neck of the fibula
    B. The lateral malleolus lies inferior and posterior to the medial malleolus
    C. The upper end of fibula ossifies at one year
    D. The tibial tuberosity and medial malleolus may appear as separate centers
    E. The upper end of epiphysis fuses at 16-18 years

41. **Joints and their types:**
    A. Superior tibiofibular joint—fibrous joint
    B. Inferior tibiofibular joint—synovial joint
    C. Ankle joint—saddle joint
    D. Calcaneocuboid joint—hinge joint
    E. Subtalar joint—synovial

42. **Ankle joint ligaments:**
    A. The posterior component of the deltoid ligament blends with the spring ligament
    B. The deltoid ligament is attached to the lateral malleolus
    C. The posterior tibiotalar ligament attaches to the medial tubercle of talus
    D. The anterior talofibular ligament attaches to the neck of the talus
    E. The tibiocalcaneal ligament is attached to the sustentaculum tali

43. **Muscles of leg and their attachment:**
    A. Tibialis anterior—first metatarsal base
    B. Peroneus brevis—third metatarsal
    C. Personal longus—first metatarsal
    D. Plantaris—calcaneus
    E. Popliteus—lateral tibial condyle

44. **Foot:**
    A. Plantar flexion is mainly produced by gastrocnemius
    B. Dorsiflexion is produced by tibialis anterior only
    C. The talus has no muscular attachments
    D. Talus is the largest tarsal bone
    E. Calcaneal axis is directed laterally

45. **Foot:**
    A. Subtalar joint is imaged optimally with oblique views in external rotation
    B. Calcaneonavicular coalition is best seen in oblique view with internal rotation
    C. Talocalcaneal coalition is diagnosed by posterior tangential view
    D. Coronal CT is necessary for subtalar joint evaluation
    E. Ultrasound can evaluate plantar fascia

46. **Foot:**
    A. Bohler's angle is > 40 degrees in crush fracture of calcaneum
    B. Calcaneal pitch should be less than 30 degrees
    C. Heel pad thickness is less than 23 mm in females
    D. Midline of foot should make an axis of 15 degrees with the axis of talus
    E. The lines of talonavicular joint and between navicular and first cuneiform should be parallel

47. **Accessory ossicles:**
    A. Sesamoid in flexor hallucis longus is the most common sesamoid
    B. Os peroneum is seen in peroneus longus tenson, in 20%
    C. Os vesalinium is found under tibialis posterior
    D. Bipartite navicular bone is the common congenital variation
    E. Bony bridge between calcaneum and cuboid is common

48. **Accessory ossicles:**
    A. Os trigonum—separate ossification for posterior surface of talus
    B. Os subtibiale—accessory ossification under lateral malleolus
    C. Os tibiale externum—5%, for navicular tuberosity
    D. Sesamoid is seen in tibialis anterior, over medial cuneiform
    E. Sesamoid in tibialis posterior is seen in 25%

49. **Causes of tarsal tunnel syndrome:**
    A. Gout
    B. Varicose veins
    C. Ganglia
    D. Accessory muscle
    E. Neurilemmoma

50. **Intraosseus lipoma:**
    A. 10% affects calcaneum
    B. Seen in center of trigonum calcis
    C. Typical pyramidal shape
    D. MRI shows central haemorrhage
    E. Peipheral rim of fatty tissue is seen

51. **Achilles tendonitis:**
    A. There is no synovial sheath for Achilles tendon
    B. Tenosynovitis is a common presentation of Achilles tendon injury
    C. Kager's triangle of fat is seen between the tendon and distal tibia
    D. Prominent superior tuberosity of calcaneum predisposes to insertional tendinosis
    E. Haglund's syndrome involves retrocalcaneal bursitis

52. **Predisposing factors of Achilles tendon injury:**
    A. Pes cavus
    B. Tibia vara
    C. Forefoot varus
    D. Shin splint
    E. Tight hamstrings

53. **Rupture of Achilles tendon:**
    A. Sustained high muscular activity is worse than intermittent athletic activity
    B. Women are more commonly affected
    C. Tear at the site of insertion of Achilles tendon
    D. Caused by violent plantar flexion
    E. Tendon gap is not felt in chronic tear

54. **Associations of Achilles tendon rupture:**
    A. Rheumatoid arthritis
    B. Gout
    C. Renal failure
    D. Hyperthyroidism
    E. Diabetes

55. **Achilles tendon rupture:**
    A. Plain X-ray is not useful in diagnosis
    B. Obliteration of Kagel's fat pad although not seen in all, is specific
    C. MRI is done only in clinically equivocal tears
    D. The tendon is thickened only in partial tear but not in complete tear
    E. Extent of the retraction of tendon ends is essential for surgery

56. **Morton's neuroma:**
    A. More common in men
    B. Seen between heads of first and second metatarsal
    C. Tenderness on lateral compression
    D. Plantar digital nerve is involved
    E. Bursitis is associated

57. **Morton's neuroma:**
    A. No contrast enhancement is seen
    B. Fat suppressed T2 weighted image is best for detection of Morton's neuroma
    C. Produced by compression of digital nerve against inter-metatarsal ligament
    D. The nerve undergoes degeneration
    E. Plantar neuromas have high signal in T2W images

58. **Features of diabetic foot:**
    A. Neuropathic joints
    B. Cellulitis
    C. Vasculitis
    D. Sinuses
    E. Osteomyelitis

59. Diabetic foot:
   A. Bone scan is not sensitive for chronic osteomyelitis
   B. Bone scan can differentiate osteomyelitis and neuropathic changes
   C. Ultrasound is sensitive than plain X-ray in detecting periosteal reaction
   D. Acute osteomyelitis is more commonly seen in diabetes than chronic osteomyelitis
   E. MRI shows periosteal reaction within a few hours of onset

ANSWERS

1. **A-F, B-F, C-F, D-T, E-T**
Causes of soft tissue calcification
Vascular causes—aging, atherosclerosis, Mönckeberg's sclerosis, DM, renal failure, hyperparathyroidism, phleboliths, venous edema.
Metabolic—hypercalcemia, hyperparathyroidism, renal failure, gout, pseudo, pseudo-pseudohypoparathyroidism
Infections—cysticercosis, guinea worm, Loa loa, armillifer, TB, leprosy
Connective tissue disorders—Scleroderma, dermatomyositis, CPPD, FOP, EDS, tumoral calcinosis, calcinosis universalis.

2. **A-T, B-T, C-T, D-F, E-T**
Neurologic disease, chronic venous insufficiency, myositis ossificans, parosteal osteosarcoma and extraskeletal osteosarcoma are other causes of soft tissue ossification.

3. **A-F, B-F, C-T, D-T, E-F**
The name is a misnomer. There is no inflammation and the primary process is in the interstitium. The muscle fibers are intact, thus differentiating it from sarcoma. Elbow, thighs, buttocks, shoulder, calf, hand and jaws are affected in that order. Both the medial and lateral sides of the elbow are affected. The exact source of the osteoblasts is not known. Theories include origin from damaged periosteum or from pluripotent stem cells.

4. **A-F, B-T, C-F, D-T, E-F**
The characteristic appearance is a rim or shell of ossification with a lucent center and the lesion is clearly separated from the underlying bone. Periostitis is formed in 10 days. Lacy new bone is formed in 6-8 weeks and mature bone is deposited in 5-6 months. There are three zones in the lesion, a central fibroblasts, haemorrhage and necrosis, intermediate osteoblasts and immature bone and peripheral mature trabeculae. Maturation is centripetal progressing from periphery to center.

5. **A-F, B-T, C-T, D-T, E-T**
The main differential diagnoses of myositis ossificans are parosteal osteosarcoma, periosteal osteosarcoma, osteoma, chondroma and osteochondroma. Parosteal osteosarcoma has a less dense and poorly circumscribed periphery, with calcification in center and base, rapidly growing, with an incomplete lucency between lesion and cortex because of attachment, predominantly in metaphysis. Periosteal osteosarcoma is in diaphysis, has cortical thickening, spiculated osteoid matrix and denser from periphery to base.

Osteoma is seen as localised osseous excrescence from cortex. In osteochondroma there is continuity between the medulla and cortex of the lesion and the underlying bone. Chondroma produces excavation of bone and rings of arcs type of chondroid calcification.

6. **A-F, B-F, C-T, D-F, E-F**
   Weavers bottom is ischial bursitis. Housemaids knee—prepatellar bursitis, Clergymans knee—infrapatellar bursitis.

7. **A-F, B-T, C-F, D-T, E-T**
   Pellegrini-Stieda disease is calcification of the medial collateral ligament which is seen as arcuate or curvilinear calcification adjacent to the medial collateral ligament. Calcification of the stylohyoid ligament is called Eagle syndrome, this produces pain, dysphagia, abnormalities in taste sensation and lump in throat. It is caused by trauma, surgery or DISH (diffuse idiopathic skeletal hyperostasis. Achilles tendon can also calcify at its body.

8. **A-F, B-T, C-T, D-T, E-T**
   Florid reactive periostitis is also called bizarre parosteal osteo-chondromatous proliferation or pseudomalignant myositis ossificans of hand or fibro-osseous pseudotumour of digits. It is seen in proximal and middle phalanges of hand. It is seen as a soft tissue masss with calcification or ossification, with extensive periosteal reaction or cortical destruction. The initial event is believed to be trauma, which induces haemorrhagic subperiosteal proliferation. This can be contained within periosteum, producing periostitis and incorporated into cortex, remodelling the bone and producing a broad-based protuberance producing pain. Or it can breach the periosteum, producing a lobular lesion attached to cortex with incomplete ossification and calcification, called bizarre osteochondromatous proliferation, which is painless.

9. **A-T, B-F, C-F, D-F, E-T, F-T**
   Cysticercosis, Dracunculus, Loa loa, Armillifer, hydatid and schistosomiasis are the common parasites causing soft tissue calcification

10. **A-F, B-F, C-F, D-T, E-T**
    The etiology is unknown but majority have inborn error of phosphate metabolism. It is usually autosomal recessive but dominant variants are also seen. Seen around large joints and in 2nd or 3rd decade. It is usually painless. Restriction of joint movement, ulceration and infection are recognised complications.

11. **A-F, B-T, C-F, D-F, E-T**
    The serum calcium is normal but phosphate and ESR are elevated. Treatment is dietary restriction of calcium and phosphorus and

phosphate-binding antacids. Surgery is reserved for nonresponding cases.

12. **A-F, B-F, C-T, D-F, E-F**

Cysticercosis is acquired by ingestion of food contaminated with ova of the *Taenia solium* (unlike the tapeworm infection). The calcification is parallel to the direction of muscle fibres and common in the limbs and brain. Armiller armillatus calcification are crescentic and similar to cysticerus in end on view, but they are commonly seen in the trunks. Guinea worm infection is by a female worm. It produces coiled calcification, similar to that of *Loa loa* infection, which is usually better seen in the hand and feet.

13. **A-F, B-F, C-T, D-T, E-T**

Fibrodysplasia ossificans progressiva is an autosomal dominant disease, with extensive calcification in the perimuscular fascia and not the muscles. Muscles are affected secondarily by pressure atrophy. The earliest changes are dysplastic changes in the first metatarsal and cervical vertebral bodies. The extensive soft tissue calcification causes severe restriction of movement and eventually results in respiratory compromise. Other causes include starvation due to TMJ and masseter ossification and pneumonia.

14. **A-T, B-F, C-T, D-T, E-T**

The disease usually begins in the neck, progressions from cranial to caudal, from axial to appendicular from dorsal to ventral. The disease has erratic exacerbations and remissions.

15. **A-T, B-T, C-T, D-T, E-F**

16. **A-T, B-F, C-T, D-T, E-T**

Renal osteodystrophy, hypoparathyroidism and hyperparathyroidism are other causes.

17. **A-T, B-T, C-T, D-T, E-T**

Metastatic calcification is deposition of calcium in normal tissues, due to raised Calcium phosphate product.

Dystrophic calcification is deposition of calcium in pathological tissues, with normal calcium and phosphorus levels.

18. **A-F, B-T, C-T, D-F, E-T**

Baker's cyst is seen as a soap bubble like cystic lesion arising in the posterior aspect of the knee, arising from the medial head of gastrocnemius muscle tendon. Neuromas may be seen as well-defined cystic lesions, showing acoustic enhancement. Colour and power Doppler are useful in evaluation of vascularity of a lesion and is better than gadolinium-enhanced MRI . Ultrasound is also an adjunct to MRI in assessment of soft tissue lesions, where high signal may not always indicate a cystic mass and the vascularity may not be assessed by MRI. The staging of a mass by MRI should always precede biopsy because (1) MRI stages the mass accurately and predicts the best way of excising the mass and best needle track. Wrong biopsy technique without MRI may result extensive seeding. (2) Postbiopsy changes make MRI evaluation of tumour difficult. Follow-up scans, for masses, should preferably be using the same modality, technique and sequences.

19. **A-T, B-T, C-T, D-T, E-T, F-T**
Although MRI is the best modality for evaluation of tendinopathy, ultrasound can also provided useful information. Tears are diagnosed by presence of fluid in and around the tendon. Dynamic assessment is possible and correlation with patients symptoms can be made. Ultrasound is useful in the diagnosis of conditions like patellar tendinosis, Achilles tendon rupture, supraspinatus tears, tennis and golfers elbow and carpal tunnel syndrome.

20. **A-T, B-F, C-T, D-T, E-F**
Presence of abnormal striations, or hemorrhage or separation suggests injury. Ultrasound is also good for detection of foreign bodies. It can detect metal fragment > 0.5 cm, wood > 0.7 mm, glass > 2 mm and plastic > 4 mm.

21. **A-T, B-T, C-T, D-T, E-T**
Causes of carpal tunnel syndrome:
RA, scleroderma, SLE, SNSA, dermatomyelitis, polymyalgia rheumatica, infections, hemophilia, amyloidosis, myxedema, acromegaly, hyperparathyroidism, DM, pregnancy, oral contraceptives, gynaecologic surgery, osteoarthritis, pyridoxine deficiency, Paget's, idiopathic.

22. **A-T, B-T, C-T, D-T, E-T**
Leukemia, myeloma and metastasis destroy bone and produce hypercalcemia.
Hyperparathyroidism, hypervitaminosis D, milk alkali syndrome, sarcoidosis and renal osteodystrophy are common causes of hypercalcemia producing soft tissue calcification.

23. **A-T, B-F, C-T, D-T, E-T**
Atherosclerosis is the common cause.
Mönckeberg's disease produces sclerosis in the tunica media.
Atherosclerosis involves the tunica intima.

24. **A-F, B-T, C-T, D-T, E-F**
Paget's does not produce soft tissue calcification.
Other causes are pseudo-pseudohypoparathyroidism, pseudogout and diabetes mellitus. Sarcoidosis causes hypercalcemia.

25. **A-T, B-T, C-T, D-T, E-T**
   High signal in muscle can be due to infection and inflammation such as necrotizing fasciitis/polymyositis dermatomyositis/ edema/ tumours/rhabdomyolysis, including metabolic abnormalities, myopathies, injuries/traumatic denervation.

26. **A-T, B-T, C-F, D-T, E-T**
   Diabetic muscular infarction is seen in uncontrolled IDDM. The mechanism is believed to be hypoxic reperfusion injury. Initially, there is thromboembolic event which causes ischemia of muscle groups. When reperfused, the muscle becomes edematous and reactive free radicals are released which worsen the edema and inflammation. It is bilateral, a mass may be felt. It is frequently recurrent.

27. **A-F, B-F, C-T, D-T, E-F**
   Muscles are hypertrophied. Usually, iso intense to muscle in T1, (may be hyperintense due to haemorrhage), hyperintense in T2. Contrast enhancement can be seen in non-necrotic areas. Edema can be seen in subcutaneous, subfascial and intermuscular planes.

28. **A-F, B-T, C-F, D-T, E-F**
   Tennis leg was originally thought to be secondary to plantaris rupture, but now thought to be due to rupture of medial head of gastrocnemius.
   Tennis elbow—lateral epicondylitis, common extensor origin.
   Golfers elbow—medial epicondylitis, common flexor origin.
   Runners knee—chondromalacia patellae
   Shin splints—can be anterior or posterior, tibialis anterior and posterior insertion.

29. **A-F, B-F, C-T, D-F, E-T**
   1 ml is enough. Tendons are hypoechoic, fibrillar with echogenic septae.

30. **A-T, B-T, C-T, D-T, E-F**
   Tennis leg is pain in midcalf, beginning with a sudden pop, following sports or running·or climbing stairs. Rupture of gastrocnemius occurs at myotendinous junction. Fluid between aponeurosis of medial head of gastrocnemius and soleus indicates tear of the medial head. The same symptoms can be produced by rupture of soleus or plantaris.

31. **A-T, B-T, C-F, D-F, E-T**
   Muscle hernia is a very rare condition and is due to a fascial defect, especially at sites of perforating vessels. The fascial defect should not be closed, because it will cause compartmental syndrome.

Treatment is just reassurance or fascial grafts. Ultrasound will show the herniated muscle, which is usually less echogenic than normal muscle (probably atrophy). Spoke-like appearance can be seen due to pinching of echogenic fibrous septa due to herniation.

32. **A-T, B-F, C-T, D-T, E-T**
Plantar fasciitis, other seronegative diseases, tumours and avascular necrosis are other causes of pain in the heel.

33. **A-T, B-T, C-F, D-T, E-T**

34. **A-T, B-T, C-T, D-T, E-T**
Forefoot pain is pain at the metatarsal regions. Other causes are stress fractures, ganglia, calluses, septic arthritis, rheumatoid arthritis, osteoarthritis, turf toe, osteomyelitis, plantar plate disruption, tumours.

35. **A-F, B-T, C-F, D-T, E-T**
Pain is characteristic in the anteromedial aspect of calcaneum. In acute stage the pain begins at the site of origin of plantar fascia and it migrates distally in chronic stages. Pain in exacerbated by dorsiflexion of foot. Pain and stiffness are worst in the morning.

36. **A-F, B-T, C-F, D-F, E-F**
Plantar calcaneal spur is not pathognomonic. Heel pad thickening is another nonspecific feature. Bone scan shows high uptake in region of calcaneus. Normal plantar fascia measures up to 3 mm and in fasciitis it is up to 7 mm. The thickening is more marked at the site of insertion to calcaneus and there is high signal in plantar fascia and adjacent soft tissue. The thickening is fusiform, unlike fibromatosis where it is nodular.

37. **A-T, B-T, C-F, D-T, E-F**
Freiberg's infraction involves osteonecrosis, fractures and collapse of 2nd or 3rd metatarsal head. In early stages there is low signal in T1 and high signal in T2 and in late stages there is low signal in both, due to sclerosis.

38. **A-T, B-F, C-T, D-F, E-F**
Talus is mainly supplied by tarsal canal artery, a branch of posterior tibial artery from the medial aspect of tarsal canal. This anastomoses with branches from dorsalis pedis artery and peronal artery from the lateral aspect of the tarsal canal. Preservation of deltoid branch of the tarsal canal artery is essential for preventing avascular necrosis.

39. **A-F, B-T, C-F, D-T, E-T**
Tarsal tunnel syndrome is an entrapment neuropathy due to compression of the posterior tibial nerve by flexor retinaculum,

posterior and inferior to the medial malleolus. The posterior tibial nerve is compressed before it divides into medial and lateral plantar nerves.

40. **A-T, B-T, C-F, D-T, E-T**
Tibia—upper end—at birth; fibular upper end—3-4 year; fuse at 16-18 years
Tibia lower end—1 year; fibular lower end—1 year; fuse at 15-17 years
Medial malleolus—7 years; tibial tuberosity—10 years.

41. **A-F, B-F, C-F, D-F, E-F**
Superior tibiofibular joint is a synovial joint and inferior is a fibrous joint.
Ankle—Hinge; calcaneocuboid—saddle; subtalar—fibrous.

42. **A-F, B-F, C-T, D-T, E-T**
Medial Side—Deltoid ligament—From medial malleolus—three insertions
1. Tibionavicular (navicular tuberosity), 2. tibiocalcaneal (sustentaculum tali of calcaneus), 3. posterior tibiotalar (medial tubercle of talus), the anterior aspect of this ligament blends with the spring ligament.
Lateral side—Three ligaments—From lateral malleolus: 1. Anterior talofibular (talar neck), 2. calcaneofibular (tubercle in calcaneum), 3. posterior talofibular (posterior process of talus).

43. **A-T, B-F, C-T, D-T, E-F**
Tibialis anterior—first metatarsal base; tibialis posterior—bases of 2,3,4 metatarsal
Peroneus longus—I metatarsal, medial cuneiform; Peroneus brevis—5 metatarsal
Peroneus tertius—shaft of 5th metatarsal.
Plantaris—calcaneus, vestigial; Popliteus—lateral femoral condyle
Extensor hallucis longus—base of distal phalanx of 1 toe
Extensor digitorum longus—base of distal phalanges of lateral four toes
Flexor hallucis longus and digitorum longus—base of distal phalanges of 1 and 2,3,4,5 toes.

44. **A-T, B-F, C-T, D-F, E-T**
Plantar flexion—posterior compartment muscles, mainly gastrocnemius and soleus.
Dorsiflexion—anterior compartment muscles
Calcaneum is the largest tarsal bone with its axis lateral, upwards, and forwards.

45. A-F, B-T, C-T, D-T, E-T
Subtalar joint oblique with internal rotation, coronal CT. Calcaneo-navicular—oblique with internal rotation. Talocalcaneal— medial oblique, lateral, posterior oblique.

46. A-F, B-T, C-F, D-T, E-T
Bohler's angle—Two lines. I—anterior lip of anterior surface of calcaneus to the posterior lip of posterior surface and II—posterior lip of posterior articular surface to the posterosuperior surface of calcaneum—28-40 degrees. Reduced in crush fractures.
Calcaneal pitch—angle between the line along posterior surface of calcaneus and horizontal. Abnormal arch formation if more than 30 degrees.
Heel pad thickness is less than 21.5 mm in females and 23 m in males.

47. A-F,B-T,C-F, D-T, E-T
Flexor hallucis brevis sesamoid is the most common. OS perneum—in peroneus longus; OS vesalinium—peroneus brevis.

48. A-T, B-F, C-T, D-T, E-T
OS trigonum is seen in 8% and bilateral in majority. OS subtibiale is seen underneath the medial malleolus, os subfibulare is seen underneath the lateral malleolus.

49. A-F, B-T, C-T, D-T, E-T
Trauma, rheumatoid arthritis flat foot, valgus foot, dislocations, tumours/bony prominences/vascular plexus in tarsal tunnel are other causes.

50. A-T, B-T, C-T, D-T, E-T
Intraosseous lipoma and simple bone cyst are typically seen in the center of trigonum and have pyramidal shape. The lesion can be diffusely hyperintense in T1 and T2 or can show central haemorrhage and a peripheral rind of fatty tissue.

51. A-T, B-F, C-T, D-T, E-T
Tenosynovitis is not seen in the absence of tendon sheath. Prominent superior tuberosity, inappropriate shoe are causes of insertional tendinosis. Insertional tendinosis, retrocalcaneal bursitis and superificial Achilles bursitis are features of Haglund's syndrome.

52. A-T, B-T, C-T, D-F, E-T

53. A-F, B-F, C-F, D-F, E-T
Intermittent athletic activity in unconditioned persons, slippery surfaces, and violent dorsiflexion of foot are predisposing causes. Men are more commonly affected and can be bilateral. Teat is at

approximately 2-6 cm from the insertion and is due to poor vascular supply and strong rotation of gastrocnemius and soleus. Tendon gap is seen in acute tear but not in chronic tear where fibrosis and scarring replace the tear.

54. **A-T, B-T, C-T, D-T, E-T,**
Steroids are an iatrogenic cause.

55. **A-F, B-F, C-T, D-F, E-T**
Plain X-ray can show obliteration of the Kagel's fat pad between the tendon and calcaneum. This is not specific as this can be seen in tumours and accesosory muscles. Clinical examination is negative in 25%. MRI should be done if the clinical diagnosis is equivocal. The tendon is thickened and shows high signal in partial tear. In tear, the ends are retracted and thickened with high signal. MRI is essential for deciding if the ends can be approximated or graft is required.

56. **A-F, B-F, C-T, D-T, E-T**
It is more common in women. The most common location is in between the heads of 3rd, 4th metatarsals or between 2nd, 3rd metatarsals. Mid foot pain radiating to toes and numbness of are characteristic features.

57. **A-F, B-F, C-T, D-T, E-T**
Lesion is hypointense in T and T2. Better detection in T1 images due to good contrast with high signal fat. Contrast enhancement occurs. Fat suppressed contrast enhanced images are optimal for detection. Theories of formation include compression of nerve against intermetatarsal ligament or by bursa or vascular ischemia and the lesion is made up of fibrosis and nerve degeneration. Unlike Marton's neuroma, plantar neuroma has high signal in T2.

58. **A-T, B-T, C-T, D-T, E-T**
Diabetic foot is a combination of all the above with ulcers and tissues necrosis.

59. **A-T, B-F, C-T, D-T, E-T**
Bone scan takes 7-10 days to become positive in osteomyelitis. Ultrasound is more sensitive. MRI is the most sensitive with good soft tissue contrast. Ultrasound is very useful for detecting fluid collections. Both osteomyelitis and neuropathic joints show high uptake.

10 Bone and Soft Tissue Tumours

1. **Lucent bone lesion with calcification:**
   A. Lipoma
   B. Ganglion
   C. Bone infarction
   D. Osteomyelitis
   E. Eosinophilic granuloma

2. **Subarticular lucent lesion:**
   A. Pigmented villonodular synovitis
   B. Osteonecrosis
   C. Tuberculosis
   D. Benign fibrous histiocytoma
   E. Unicameral bone cyst

3. **Expansile lytic lesion:**
   A. Fibrous dysplasia
   B. Hemophilia
   C. Brown tumour
   D. Hydatid
   E. Tuberculosis

4. **Lucent lesion with eccentric expansion:**
   A. Enchondroma
   B. Adamantinoma
   C. Chondromyxoid fibroma
   D. Eosinophilic granuloma
   E. Giant cell tumour

5. **Ill-defined lucent lesion in medulla:**
   A. Ewing's
   B. Osteomyelitis
   C. Myeloma
   D. Fibrosarcoma
   E. Eosinophilic granuloma

6. **Differential diagnosis for well-defined lucent lesion without sclerosis, no expansion:**
   A. Myeloma
   B. Metastasis
   C. Brown tumour
   D. Chondroblastoma
   E. Fibrous dysplasia

7. **Age distribution of tumours in decades:**
   A. Simple bone cyst 3-4
   B. ABC 2-3
   C. Ewing's 1-2
   D. Osteosarcoma parosteal 2-3
   E. Lymphoma 2-3

8. **Age distribution of common bone tumours:**
   A. Osteoid osteoma 2-3
   B. Osteoma 2-3
   C. Osteoblastoma 2-3
   D. Chondroblastoma 1-2
   E. Hemangioma 1-2

9. **Following tumours are seen in seventh decade:**
   A. Hemangioma
   B. Osteosarcoma
   C. Lymphoma
   D. Chordoma
   E. Fibrosarcoma

10. **Common diaphyseal tumours:**
    A. Enchondroma
    B. Chondromyxoid fibroma
    C. Osteoid osteoma
    D. Adamantinoma
    E. Eosinophilic granuloma

11. **Common causes of metaphyseal tumours:**
    A. Fibrosarcoma
    B. Chondroblastoma
    C. Benign fibrous histiocytoma
    D. Fibrosarcoma
    E. Chondrosarcoma

12. **Moth-eaten pattern of destruction is seen in:**
    A. Lymphoma   B. Plasmacytoma
    C. Leukemia   D. Chondrosarcoma
    E. Osteomyelitis

13. **Osteoblastoma:**
    A. Common in vertebra than peripheral skeleton
    B. Majority are in diaphysis
    C. Painful and expansile
    D. Uniformly benign
    E. Recurrence in 10%

14. **Osteoblastoma:**
    A. Always more than 1.5 cm
    B. A common cause of painful scoliosis
    C. Majority respond to salicylates
    D. In spine most common location is the body
    E. Ossified matrix

15. **Well-defined lucent lesion with sclerotic rim:**
    A. Eosinophilic granuloma
    B. Fibrous dysplasia
    C. Chondroblastoma
    D. Brodie's abscess
    E. Hemangioma

16. **Osteoblastoma:**
    A. Periosteal reaction seen
    B. Disuse osteoporosis is a common feature
    C. Sclerotic rim is present
    D. Can be purely sclerotic in spine
    E. Soft tissue component absent

17. **Osteoid osteoma:**
    A. Always less than 1.5 cm
    B. Pathologically easily distinguishable from osteoblastoma
    C. 10-20 years
    D. Uncommon before five years
    E. Pain worse at night

18. **Osteoid osteoma:**
    A. Posterior elements of spine are more commonly involved than anterior body
    B. Diaphyseal in long bones
    C. Commonly nidus is seen within the cortex
    D. Laminated periosteal reaction
    E. Cortex is thickened

19. **Ewing's sarcoma:**
    A. Bony metastasis
    B. 25% arise from metaphysis
    C. Head and neck tumor has worst prognosis
    D. Periosteal reaction is seen only after the permeative pattern appears
    E. Has concentric growth pattern

20. **Osteoid osteoma:**
    A. Percutaneous ethanol injection is very effective
    B. Nidus enhances in contrast enhanced CT
    C. Bone scan shows central cold area surrounded by hot area
    D. High signal intensity in T2W images
    E. Isointense to muscle in T1

21. **Osteoma:**
    A. Associated with Turcot's syndrome
    B. Common from the inner table of skull
    C. Most common in the frontal sinus
    D. Less than 2 cm
    E. Homogeneously sclerotic

22. **Osteofibrous dysplasia:**
    A. Seen 10-20 years
    B. Almost exclusively occurs in tibia
    C. Anterior cortex predominantly affected
    D. Has sclerotic margin
    E. Surgery to prevent deformity

23. **Giant cell tumour:**
    A. Presents before epiphyseal closure
    B. Centrally located in the bone
    C. Surrounded by thin sclerotic margin
    D. Associated with periosteal reaction
    E. Most common around the shoulder joint

24. **Chordoma:**
    A. Arises from arachnoid cap cells
    B. Most common in the sacrococcygeal region
    C. L3 is the common lumbar vertebra involved
    D. Physalipharous cells are pathognomonic
    E. Rapid growth is characteristic

25. **Chordoma:**
    A. Calcification is very common
    B. Soft tissue mass is essential for diagnosis
    C. Well-defined bone destruction
    D. In sacrum, the soft tissue component extends posteriorly
    E. Men more commonly affected

26. **Primary bone lymphoma:**
    A. Usually Hodgkin's lymphoma
    B. Metaphysis is the commonly affected portion
    C. Flat bones not affected
    D. Biphasic distribution of age
    E. Low-grade

27. Lymphoma:
A. All cases have intratumoral fibrosis
B. No sclerosis is seen
C. Moth-eaten pattern is most common
D. Soft tissue invasion late
E. Vertebral lesion excludes primary lymphoma

28. Ewing's sarcoma:
A. Second common malignant bone tumour in children after osteosarcoma
B. Can take origin from subperiosteal region
C. Peak age is between 1-5 years
D. Fever is a common presentation
E. Raised ESR

29. Ewing's sarcoma:
A. Soft tissue mass with preservation of soft tissue planes
B. Flat bone Ewing's are more sclerotic
C. Sunburst spiculation is sparse and delicate
D. Dynamic MRI is not of any use in assessment of Ewing's
E. Bone is the most common organ to which metastasis happens

30. Differential diagnosis for Ewing's:
A. Osteomyelitis   B. Lymphoma
C. Neuroblastoma   D. Eosinophilic granuloma
E. Osteosarcoma

31. Osteoid osteoma:
A. Angio shows intense vascularity
B. Nidus is always lucent
C. Scoliosis is seen with convexity towards the lesion
D. If located subperiosteally, there is more sclerosis than other locations
E. Spontaneous regression recognised

32. Intra-articular osteoid osteoma:
A. Early presentation
B. Osteoarthritis
C. No sclerosis
D. Joint space narrowed
E. Most common in hip joint

33. Eosinophilic granuloma:
A. Expansion of medullary cavity is seen
B. Pathological fracture is common
C. Ill-defined margin is the common feature
D. Lamellar periosteal reaction
E. Loss of tubulation at the metaphysis

34. **Association of erosion of the ilium and adjacent soft tissue is seen in:**
    A. Plasmacytoma
    B. Haemophilia
    C. Chordoma
    D. Hodgkin's disease
    E. Fibrosarcoma

35. **Ameloblastoma of jaw:**
    A. Symphysis menti is characteristically involved
    B. Root resorption is seen
    C. Multilocular cystic appearance is seen
    D. Sclerosis of bone trabeculae
    E. Mandible is more commonly involved than maxilla

36. **Ribs are commonly involved in:**
    A. Chondroblastoma
    B. Osteoid osteoma
    C. Osteochondroma
    D. Fibrous dysplasia
    E. Nonossifying fibroma

37. **The following are malignant round cell tumours of bone:**
    A. Lymphoma
    B. Ewing's
    C. PNET
    D. Myeloma
    E. Neuroblastoma

38. **Primary malignancies with increased uptake in bone scan:**
    A. Meningioma
    B. Lung
    C. Neuroblastoma
    D. Hepatoma
    E. Glioblastoma multiforme

39. **Multiple myeloma:**
    A. Associated with Vater syndrome
    B. Gallium scan shows uptake
    C. Doughnut sign is seen
    D. Amyloid causes increased uptake in bone scan
    E. Multiple myeloma shows hypointensity both T1 and T2 after treatment

40. **Multiple myeloma:**
    A. In any juxta-articular location, crosses the joint, to involve multiple joint surfaces
    B. Sclerosis is seen in 10% of cases
    C. Sclerosis is more common than lytic type occurs in an older population
    D. Extramedullary plasmacytoma converts to myeloma more often than solitary plasmacytoma
    E. The alkaline phosphatase cannot be a differentiating factor between osteoporosis circumscripta and solitary plasmacytoma

41. Features in favour of myeloma than metastasis:
   A. Erosion of pedicles
   B. Generalized osteoporosis
   C. Elevated serum alkaline phosphatase
   D. Soft tissue mass
   E. Involvement of adjacent disc space

42. Ewing's sarcoma:
   A. Tumor made up of round cells
   B. Saucerisation is a characteristic feature
   C. Onion peel appearance is pathognomonic
   D. Codman's triangle is seen
   E. Eccentric location

43. Osteosarcoma:
   A. Bone scan underestimates the medullary involvement
   B. MRI is the best for assessing tumour extent in marrow
   C. Lung metastasis shows increased uptake in bone scan
   D. Pneumothorax is common in lung metastasis
   E. CT chest should be done before treatment

44. Osteosarcoma of jaw:
   A. Older age group than conventional osteosarcoma
   B. Majority are chondroblastic
   C. Higher grade than routine tumours
   D. Sclerotic if mandible is affected
   E. More periosteal reaction if lesion in maxilla

45. Telangiectactic osteosarcoma:
   A. Fluid-fluid levels seen in MRI
   B. Doughnut sign in bone scan
   C. Diaphyseal
   D. Permeative pattern of destruction
   E. Common in vertebrae

46. Parosteal osteosarcoma:
   A. May be confused with myositis ossificans
   B. Pre-existing Paget's disease makes the prognosis worse
   C. CT is essential for showing intramedullary extension
   D. 50% occur in the distal half of the femur
   E. Commonly arise from paraosteal chondroma

47. Osteosarcoma:
   A. Most common malignant bone tumour
   B. Uncommon before 10 years
   C. Second peak in fifty years
   D. 75% of lesions are seen around the knee
   E. Majority have chondroblastic pathology

48. **Osteosarcoma:**
    A. Does not affect epiphysis
    B. Large than 5 cm at presentation
    C. Lymphatic spread seen
    D. Periosteal reaction is the earliest finding
    E. Geographical pattern

49. **Osteosarcoma:**
    A. Sunburst periosteal reaction is specific
    B. Codman's triangle indicates rapid soft tissue growth
    C. Purely lytic lesion shows geographical pattern
    D. MRI is best for assessing extraosseous spread of tumour
    E. CT is best for assessing ossification in matrix

50. **Parosteal osteosarcoma:**
    A. Metaphyseal location
    B. Periosteal reaction is commonly seen
    C. Well-defined outer margin is characteristic
    D. More vascular than osteosarcoma in angiography
    E. Younger age group than osteosarcoma

51. **Chondrosarcoma, conventional:**
    A. More common in females
    B. Common 5th decade
    C. Proximal aspects of bone are commonly involved than the distal part
    D. Pathological fractures are seen in 50%
    E. Scapula is the most common flat bone affected

52. **Secondary osteosarcomas are seen in:**
    A. Radiation
    B. Fibrous dysplasia
    C. Avascular necrosis
    D. Osteogenesis imperfecta
    E. Osteomyelitis

53. **Sarcomas in Paget's disease:**
    A. Fibrosarcoma is the most common tumour
    B. 1% malignant conversion
    C. Not seen in monostotic disease
    D. Spine is not involved
    E. Low uptake in Paget's disease is suggestive

54. **Bone tumours:**
    A. The most common site of giant cell tumour in spine is sacrum
    B. Benign chondroblastoma is most common in long bone metaphysis

C. The most common site in the spine for aneurysmal bone cyst is the body of vertebra
D. Nonossifying fibroma is never found in the midshaft of a long bone
E. Most common site in spine for osteoid osteoma is the neural arch

55. **Bone tumours:**
A. Cavitation is more common in secondary than peripheral primary neoplasms
B. Myeloma affects the mandible more often than secondary neoplasm
C. Pedicle destruction is more often due to myeloma than secondary neoplasm
D. Large extrapleural masses are found in myeloma
E. Myelomatosis can give rise to osteoblastic lesions

56. **Adamantinoma of long bones:**
A. Most common in the metaphysis of long bones
B. Occurs in adults aged 20-50
C. Causes severe pain
D. Associated with significant periosteal reaction
E. Satellite lesions seen

57. **Chondrosarcomas:**
A. Clear cell tumours are high-grade
B. Mesenchymal tumours are very high-grade
C. Dedifferentiated tumours are characterised by collision of two tumours
D. Dedifferentiated tumours are of low-grade
E. Myxoid tumours are intermediate type and are more common in soft tissue

58. **Chondrosarcoma:**
A. Shows ring and arcs pattern of calcification
B. Lobular architecture is characteristic
C. Endosteal scalloping
D. Majority are more than 10 cm
E. Soft tissue extension is uncommon

59. **Juxtacortical chondrosarcomas:**
A. Arise from enchondromas
B. Medullary invasion is rare in juxtacortical tumour
C. Cortical erosion is seen in juxtacortical tumour
D. No capsule is seen in juxtacortical tumour
E. High-grade tumours

60. Chondrosarcoma, conventional:
   A. Higher the grade of tumour, lesser the calcification
   B. Permeative pattern is not seen
   C. Length of endosteal scalloping is the most important feature
   D. Endosteal scalloping >2/3rd of cortex is suggestive of enchondroma than chondrosarcoma
   E. Soft tissue extension is rare

61. Types of malignancies that arise in dedifferentiated chondrosarcomas:
   A. Malignant fibrous histiocytoma
   B. Osteosarcoma
   C. Leiomyosarcoma
   D. Rhabdomyosarcoma
   E. Malignant fibrous histiocytoma

62. Parosteal osteosarcoma:
   A. More common in patients over 25 years old
   B. More common in males than females
   C. Usually arises in metaphysis
   D. Has a characteristic ill-defined margin
   E. Associated with lamellar type of periosteal reaction

63. Chondrosarcomas:
   A. CT shows low density lesion
   B. 90% of lesions show calcification in CT
   C. Higher the grade, greater the soft tissue extension
   D. Enhancement of septa is seen
   E. Rim enhancement is seen in high-grade tumours

64. Poor prognosis factors in osteosarcoma:
   A. Tumour more than 10 cm
   B. Pneumothorax
   C. Skip lesions
   D. Fracture
   E. Soft tissue mass

65. Features of juxtacortical chondrosarcoma than chondroma:
   A. Older age   B. Hair on end periosteal reaction
   C. Metaphyseal   D. Osteoblastic component
   E. Has stalk

66. Chondrosarcoma—MRI:
   A. High signal in T1 may be seen
   B. Low signal in T2 in high-grade tumours
   C. Diffuse nodular enhancement in high-grade tumours
   D. Dynamic MRI is useful for assessing grade of tumour
   E. MRI is best for assessing endosteal scalloping

67. **Chondrosarcomas and enchondromas:**
    A. More common in ribs than enchondromas
    B. Seen more in posterior aspect of ribs
    C. Enchondromas are more common in short bones
    D. Enchondromas are rare in pelvic bones
    E. Pelvic chondrosarcomas are commonly seen around triradiate cartilage

68. **Clear cell chondrosarcoma:**
    A. Seen in metaphysis
    B. Has worse prognosis than conventional
    C. Seen in 3-5 decade
    D. Constitutes 10% of chondrosarcomas
    E. Most common site is innominate bone

69. **Nonossifying fibroma:**
    A. Seen in 50% of asymptomatic boys above two years of age
    B. Seen commonly in anterior and lateral cortices
    C. More common in males
    D. Migrates to diaphysis with age
    E. Called as fibrous cortical defect if less than 3 cm

70. **Nonossifying fibroma:**
    A. Multiple nonossifying fibromas are associated with mental retardation
    B. Jaffe-Campanacci syndrome is associated with hypogonadism
    C. Pathologic fracture is common
    D. Periostitis is suggestive of aggressive lesion
    E. They always have well-defined margins

71. **Clear cell chondrosarcoma:**
    A. No calcification is seen
    B. Rind of sclerosis is characteristic
    C. Soft tissue component is common
    D. T1 is homogeneous intermediate signal
    E. T2 is heterogeneous

72. **Following are features in favour of chondrosarcoma rather than enchondroma:**
    A. More deeper scalloping
    B. Remodelling of bone
    C. Cortical thinning
    D. Uptake in bone scan
    E. Periosteal reaction

73. **Multifocal osteosarcoma:**
    A. In type I, multiple synchronous lesions, in patients above 18 years
    B. In type III, lesions are metachronous
    C. All lesions are of same size
    D. Bilaterally symmetrical
    E. All lesions are sclerotic

74. **Periosteal osteosarcoma:**
    A. Better prognosis than conventional osteosarcoma
    B. Cortex destroyed
    C. Medullary cavity involved in later stages
    D. Scalloping of cortex
    E. Diaphyseal

75. **Following are differentiating features of chondrosarcoma from chondroblastoma:**
    A. Epiphyseal involvement
    B. Older age
    C. No edema
    D. Larger
    E. T2—intermediate signal

76. **Juxtacortical chondrosarcomas:**
    A. Medullary cavity involved in later stages
    B. Affects anterior aspect of distal femoral metaphysis
    C. The cortex is thinned
    D. Seen in first and second decade
    E. Seen in innominate bone

77. **Dedifferentiated chondrosarcoma:**
    A. Can be low to high-grade
    B. High-grade lesions are low density in CT scans
    C. High-grade lesions have diffuse enhancement
    D. Common in 5th, 6th decades
    E. It is due to malignancy arising in pseudocapsule of low-grade tumour

78. **Synovial cell sarcoma:**
    A. Highest incidence is seen in the 50-70 age group
    B. Lower limb is more frequently affected than the upper limb
    C. Soft tissue calcification is seen in 25% of the cases
    D. Exposure to vinyl chloride is a predisposing factor
    E. Tendon sheaths may be the site of origin

79. **Ossifying fibroma:**
    A. Synonymous with fibrous dysplasia
    B. Anterior aspect of tibial diaphysis is the most common location
    C. Has a ground glass matrix
    D. Affects tooth-bearing portion of mandible and maxilla
    E. There is a band of sclerosis around the tumour

80. **Differential diagnosis of eccentric lytic lesion in metaphysic of a child:**
    A. Osteoid osteoma
    B. Nonossifying fibroma
    C. Brodie's abscess
    D. Chondromyxoid fibroma
    E. Chondroma

81. **Intraosseous ganglion:**
    A. Communicates with the joint
    B. Sclerotic margin
    C. Seen in metaphysis
    D. Increased uptake can be seen in bone scan
    E. Internal septations are seen in MRI

82. **Aneurysmal bone cyst:**
    A. Located in metaphysis
    B. Seen prior to epiphyseal fusion
    C. 20% have pre-existing bone pathology
    D. Pedicle of vertebra is involved commonly than the body
    E. Lie centrally in the bone
    F. Lined by endothelium

83. **Metastasis:**
    A. Healing of pathological fractures is quicker with breast and prostate metastasis
    B. Bone can be involved in metastatic disease by lymphatic spread
    C. Prostate cancer spreads to spine via the arterial system
    D. Ependymoma is the most common primary tumor to metastasise via CSF
    E. In prostate cancer, bone metastasis indicates presence of overt or cryptic lung metastasis

84. **Aneurysmal bone cyst:**
    A. Can be purely solid
    B. In bone scan, there is increased uptake in the periphery with cold center
    C. Injection of ethibloc with radiological guidance is used in recurrence of surgically proved ABC
    D. The entire lesion is very vascular in angiography
    E. Does not extend to soft tissue since it is a benign tumour

85. **Bone tumours occurring in patients less than 30 years of age:**
    A. Osteoid osteoma   B. Fibrosarcoma
    C. Ewing's sarcoma   D. Chordoma
    E. Plasmacytoma

86. **Sclerotic bone lesions:**
    A. The cortex and medulla of osteomas are continuous with the medulla of the parent bone
    B. Osteomas show gallium uptake
    C. In bone infarction there is a rim of calcification
    D. Medullary osteoid osteoma—surrounded by a rim of sclerosis
    E. Bone island—radiating spicules

87. **Chondromyxoid fibroma:**
    A. Commonly seen after the age of 50
    B. Have sclerotic rim
    C. Tibia is the most common site
    D. Calcification is never seen
    E. Located in epiphysis of long bone

88. **Spinal metastases:**
    A. The dorsal vertebra is the most common site involved
    B. The body is involved more common than posterior elements
    C. The disc height is lost in late stages of disease
    D. Breast metastasis has a predilection of L2 vertebra
    E. Spinal cord compression is produced only by an intradural lesion

89. **Metastases:**
    A. Carcinoid mets are predominantly lytic
    B. Stomach mets are sclerotic
    C. Bladder mets are calcified
    D. Breast mets are the most common sclerotic mets in a female
    E. Renal mets are sclerotic

90. **The following metastasis are purely lytic:**
    A. Head and neck cancers
    B. Adrenal
    C. Bladder
    D. Nasopharynx
    E. Hepatoma

91. **The following metastasis are purely sclerotic:**
    A. Neuroblastoma   B. Pheochromocytoma
    C. Medulloblastoma   D. Uterus
    E. Ovarian

92. **Mesenchymal chondrosarcoma:**
    A. Intermediate signal in MRI
    B. Most common in maxilla and mandible
    C. Finely stippled calcification
    D. Serpentine vessels seen in MRI
    E. Intense immediate enhancement seen

93. **Factors in favour of metastasis than primary tumour:**
    A. Diaphyseal
    B. Involvement of vertebral body
    C. No periosteal reaction
    D. No soft tissue mass
    E. No new bone formation

94. **Batson's plexus of veins:**
    A. Flow is in one direction from the caudal to cranial end
    B. Communicates with veins in spinal canal
    C. Coughing and sneezing change the flow in the veins
    D. Valves are present every 5 cm
    E. The flow is subject to direct pressure of thoracoabdominal muscles

95. **Metastasis:**
    A. In prostate carcinoma the sclerosis is due to reactive bone formation
    B. Medullary lesions are detected earlier than cortical lesions
    C. Lung cancer is the most common metastasis distal to the knee and elbows
    D. Uterine metastasis to leg spreads by retrograde venous spread
    E. Metastasis does not occur in a pre-existing Paget's disease

96. **Metastases:**
    A. Hypocalcemia is seen due to extensive bone destruction
    B. Alkaline phosphatase level is increased in serum indicates co-existing liver disease
    C. An osteolytic lesion heals by becoming sclerotic
    D. Sudden appearance of a new sclerotic lesion after treatment indicates only the appearance of a new metastasis
    E. Carcinoma prostate can heal without change in size

97. **Exuberant periosteal reaction is seen in the following metastasis:**
    A. Neuroblastoma
    B. Testis
    C. Prostate
    D. Bladder
    E. Lung

98. **Multiple myeloma:**
    A. Hypocalcemia
    B. Bence Jones proteinuria in all patients
    C. Polyclonal gamma globulin production
    D. Almost always more than 40 years
    E. Stippling in red blood cells

99. **Multiple myeloma:**
    A. Bone scan underestimates myeloma
    B. Bone scan useful for rib lesions
    C. MRI is the most sensitive
    D. Sclerosis is not seen without radiation
    E. Periosteal reaction is commonly seen

100. **Metastasis:**
    A. Solitary metastasis is more common in renal and thyroid
    B. Moth-eaten pattern of destruction is characteristic of lymphoma
    C. Soft tissue involvement is most common in colonic cancer metastasis
    D. Pathological fracture is more common in proximal femur than vertebra
    E. Pathological fracture occurs only when more than 50% of cortex is destroyed

101. **Osteochondromas:**
    A. The most common bone tumour
    B. Most common benign bone tumour
    C. 65% occur around knee and humerus
    D. 5% occur in vertebra
    E. Epiphyseal origin is common

102. **Osteochondromas:**
    A. Grow towards the joint as age progresses
    B. May grow beyond skeletal maturity
    C. Complications are directly related to size
    D. Arise secondary to irradiation
    E. The actively growing part is the cap

103. **Multiple myeloma:**
    A. Acute renal failure is the most common cause of death
    B. Nonionic contrast should be used to avoid renal failure
    C. Amyloidosis common in light chain type
    D. ESR elevated
    E. Waldenström's macroglobulinemia produces IgG

104. Multiple myeloma:
- **A.** X-rays are sensitive than bone scans
- **B.** 30% of lesions are detected only by X-rays
- **C.** In head, mandible is not affected
- **D.** Endosteal scalloping is a characteristic feature
- **E.** Can present with generalized osteoporosis

105. Eosinophilic granuloma:
- **A.** Solitary in 50% of cases
- **B.** Can be cold in radioisotope scan
- **C.** Never occurs after the age of 55
- **D.** Expansile lesions in vertebral body
- **E.** Different phases of destruction can be seen in the same lesion

106. Eosinophilic granuloma:
- **A.** Associated with diabetes mellitus
- **B.** Causes exophthalmos
- **C.** Higher incidence in women than men
- **D.** Causes aural discharge
- **E.** Causes pulmonary fibrosis

107. Hemangiomas:
- **A.** Can involve only part of vertebra
- **B.** Spinal cord compression can occur, even though it is a benign lesion
- **C.** Can be hot in bone scan
- **D.** 10% involve pedicles
- **E.** Polka dot appearance in CT

108. Differential diagnosis of coarse trabeculae in hemangioma:
- **A.** Paget's disease
- **B.** Lymphoma
- **C.** Multiple myeloma
- **D.** Eosinophilic granuloma
- **E.** Metastasis

109. Hemangioma–osseous:
- **A.** High signal intensity in more T1 and T2 images
- **B.** Majority are of capillary type
- **C.** Vertebral hemangiomas are cavernous type
- **D.** Fat is seen in vertebral hemangiomas
- **E.** The symptoms are directly correlated with the amount of fat in the lesion

110. The following bone tumours can show spontaneous regression:
- **A.** Exostosis
- **B.** Eosinophilic granuloma
- **C.** Osteoid osteoma
- **D.** Simple bone cyst
- **E.** Nonossifying fibroma

111. **Malignant fibrous histiocytoma:**
    A. More commonly seen in bone rather than soft tissue
    B. May arise from bone infarcts
    C. May be caused by radiation
    D. Most common bone tumour to complicate Paget's disease
    E. Punctate central calcification

112. **Osteochondromas:**
    A. Majority are asymptomatic
    B. Diaphyseal aclasis is autosomal dominant
    C. Presence of bursa indicates a benign process
    D. Rim enhancement around a soft tissue mass adjacent to the cartilage cap excludes a bursa
    E. Pseudoaneurysm is the most common vascular complication

113. **Hemangiomas:**
    A. In skull hemangiomas, the outer table is more expanded than the inner table
    B. Can mimic lipoma when in soft tissue
    C. Soft tissue hemangiomas associated with Klippel-Trenaunay-Weber syndrome
    D. Flow void is seen in MRI
    E. Synovial hemangioma is seen in knee

114. **Osteochondromas:**
    A. Pseudoaneurysm is common in the proximal superficial femoral artery
    B. Pedunculated osteochondromas rather than sessile osteochondromas are the common cause of pseudoaneurysm
    C. Pulsation artefacts will be seen in pseudoaneurysm
    D. Common peroneal nerve is the commonly involved nerve
    E. Atrophic changes in short head of biceps femoris indicates common personal nerve involvement

115. **Differential diagnosis of positive metacarpal sign:**
    A. Juvenile rheumatoid arthritis
    B. Sickle cell anemia
    C. Neonatal hyperthyroidism
    D. Hyperparathyroidism
    E. Multiple epiphyseal dysplasia

116. **Deformities associated with diaphyseal aclasia:**
    A. Madelung's deformity
    B. Talar slant
    C. Leg length discrepancy
    D. Valgus deformity
    E. Varus deformity

117. **Osteochondroma and malignant conversion:**
    A. 25% risk of malignancy in diaphyseal aclasia
    B. Fibrosarcoma is the most common malignancy
    C. Chondrosarcoma is common in the pelvis
    D. Biopsy should be taken at the most thickest portion of the cartilage cap
    E. More than 75% of malignant conversion takes place in the axial skeleton

118. **Indicators of malignant conversion of osteochondroma:**
    A. Unexplained pain
    B. Fracture
    C. Cartilage cap > 12 mm
    D. Lucency within cartilage
    E. Irregular osteochondral surface

119. **Simple bone cyst:**
    A. Most common in the proximal femur
    B. Appears multilocular in 25%
    C. Recurs if the patient is older than 10 years
    D. Recurs if it is in mandible
    E. Recurs after curettage in > 10%

120. **Simple bone cyst:**
    A. Eccentrically placed in cortex
    B. Lesions in the diaphysis are inactive
    C. In talus, involves the superior surface
    D. In calcaneum, the anterior margin is curvilinear
    E. The long axis of the lesion is parallel to the native bone

121. **Complications of osteochondroma:**
    A. Brachial artery pseudoaneurysm
    B. Carotid occlusion
    C. Haemothorax
    D. Synostosis
    E. Pressure erosion of bone

122. **Simple bone cyst:**
    A. The earliest finding is a small dense lesion
    B. Falling fragment sign can be seen only if there is fracture
    C. Percutaneous injection of ethibloc if recurrence after medroxy-progesterone acetate
    D. Lesions in proximal femur convert to cementifying fibroma
    E. Malignant transformation to osteosarcoma is recognized

123. **Tumours showing giant cells in pathology:**
    A. Aneurysmal bone cyst
    B. Osteosarcoma
    C. Fibrous dysplasia
    D. Osteoblastoma
    E. Chondromyxoid fibroma

124. **Differential diagnosis of soap bubble pattern in bone:**
    A. Hemangioma
    B. Fibrous dysplasia
    C. Nonossifying fibroma
    D. Desmoplastic fibroma
    E. Ewing's sarcoma

125. **Giant cell tumour:**
    A. 60% of lesions are purely lytic without septations
    B. Can cause complete vanishing of bone
    C. Occurs in the anterior aspect of calcaneum
    D. Lesions in sternum and ribs mimic metastasis
    E. Treatment results in rapid exacerbation of lytic lesion

126. **Radiation-induced sarcomas:**
    A. Latent period of at least 5 years must be allowed
    B. Osteosarcoma is the most common radiation-induced sarcoma
    C. Malignant fibrous histiocytoma is the most common soft tissue postradiation sarcoma
    D. In patients irradiated for extraosseous tumours, bone sarcomas are the most common radiation-induced tumours than extraosseous lesions
    E. Bimodal age distribution is seen for soft tissue postradiation sarcomas

127. **Giant cell tumour:**
    A. Recurrence after five years indicates malignancy
    B. Recurrence is seen in 60%
    C. Can arise in Paget's disease
    D. Distal radius tumours metastasise
    E. The only benign tumour to implant at distal site

128. **Giant cell tumours:**
    A. Metastasis does not necessarily indicate malignant giant cell tumour
    B. 10% of GCT are malignant
    C. Moth-eaten pattern indicates malignant GCT
    D. Seeding in soft tissue occurs during surgery
    E. Radiation is a predisposing factor for development

129. **Radiation-induced sarcomas:**
    A. The latent period is longer for radiation-induced soft tissue sarcomas than bone sarcomas
    B. High doses more than 50 Gy are high risk for developing subsequent cancers
    C. Tumours are more common in the center of the radiation field rather than the periphery
    D. Craniofacial lesions have grave prognosis than limb girdle lesions
    E. Chemotherapy increases the risk of second cancer

130. **Imaging of postradiation sarcomas:**
    A. MRI is the earliest indicator
    B. Soft tissue mass is the most common finding
    C. Periosteal reaction is a sensitive finding
    D. X-ray changes after five years of stability is indicative
    E. Mineralisation is suggestive

131. **Ollier's disease:**
    A. All multiple chondromas are not necessarily Ollier's disease
    B. Ollier's is asymmetrical
    C. Ollier's do not have deformity in bones
    D. 70% malignant conversion in Ollier's
    E. Ollier's is bilateral

132. **Metaphyseal involvement is common in:**
    A. Lymphoma
    B. Tuberculosis
    C. Osteoid osteoma
    D. Malignant fibrous histiocytoma
    E. Simple bone cyst

133. **Chondromyxoid fibroma:**
    A. Occurs more commonly around knee joint
    B. 30-40 years is the peak age of distribution
    C. Lesions are usually metaphyseal
    D. Irregular endosteal margin
    E. Calcification is very common

134. **Signs of recurrence of malignant tumour in MRI:**
    A. Reappearance of edema
    B. New area of high signal in T2 weighted images, with intermediate signal in T1W
    C. Change in contour of muscle
    D. Change in contour of postsurgical field
    E. Low signal in both T2 and T1

135. **Giant cell tumour:**
    A. Commonly have periosteal reaction
    B. Subarticular
    C. Occurs before epiphyseal fusion
    D. Does not affect joint space
    E. Internal septa are due to new bone formation

136. **Glomus tumours:**
    A. Painful vascular tumours
    B. Sensitive to heat
    C. Ill-defined lytic lesion of phalanx in plain films
    D. Easily detected in standard bone scan
    E. Hemangiopericytomas carry a significant risk of malignancy

137. **Chondroblastoma:**
    A. Diaphyseal location is more common than metaphysis
    B. Malignant transformation in 30%
    C. Calcification is very frequently seen
    D. Periosteal reaction is characteristic
    E. Crosses epiphysis

138. **Malignant schwannoma:**
    A. The nerve runs through the lesion
    B. Associated with rhabdomyosarcoma in Triton tumour
    C. More common in cranial than peripheral nerves
    D. Eighth nerve is the most common cranial nerve involved
    E. Recurrence very common

139. **Malignant schwannoma in neurofibromatosis:**
    A. Younger age group   B. Slow growth
    C. No metastasis   D. No sarcomatous change
    E. Difficult to resect

140. **Soft tissue neurogenic tumours:**
    A. Solitary neurofibromas are associated with NF-1
    B. Neurilemmomas are not associated with NF-1
    C. Neurilemmomas are mainly made of Schwann cells
    D. Ultrasound shows echogenic rim, due to capsule formation
    E. Ganglioneuroblastoma is most common in the sciatic nerve

141. **Bone tumours and .pathological fracture:**
    A. Prostate cancers are less likely to be fractured than breast carcinoma metastasis
    B. Radiation of the metastasis increases the risk of fracture
    C. In breast carcinoma, lytic lesions fracture more than sclerotic or mixed lesions
    D. All patients with more than 50% of cortical involvement with metastasis will develop fracture
    E. A subtrochanteric metastasis will fracture only if more than 25% of cortex is destroyed

142. **Tumours arising secondary to bone marrow transplantation:**
  A. Melanoma
  B. Carcinoma tongue
  C. Lymphoma
  D. Brain
  E. Thyroid

143. **Bone tumours:**
  A. Lesions should be more than 1 cm to be detected by X-rays
  B. Lung cancer is the most common primary tumour to present with pathological fracture
  C. Pain in metastasis is very uncommon
  D. Noras lesion refers to bizarre parosteal osteochondromatous lesion
  E. Hardcastles syndrome—association of malignant fibrous histiocytoma and medullary stenosis

144. **Fibromatosis:**
  A. Majority are multiple
  B. Low in both T1 and T2
  C. Malignant lesion
  D. Superficial lesions are more aggressive than deep lesions
  E. Can occur in bones

145. **Metastasis to muscle is seen in the following primary tumours:**
  A. Pancreas
  B. Kidney
  C. Ovary
  D. Stomach
  E. Colon

146. **Metastasis to skeletal muscle is uncommon because:**
  A. pH of muscle
  B. Mechanical destruction of tumour
  C. Absence of lymphatics
  D. Movement of muscles
  E. Lack of clearance of tumour produced lactic acid

147. **Causes of fluid-fluid level in MRI:**
  A. Aneurysmal bone cyst
  B. Adamantinoma
  C. Fibrous dysplasia
  D. Simple bone cyst
  E. Giant cell tumour

148. **Metastasis:**
    A. Hip joint is the most common joint involved in periarticular spread with intra-articular extension
    B. Pelvic muscles are the most common muscles involved in metastasis
    C. Leukemia is the most common to metastasise to synovial membrane
    D. Metastasis causes discal narrowing by producing secondary degenerative changes
    E. Direct hematogenous implantation in the disc occurs in the peripheral aspect of the discovertebral junction

149. **Tumours producing low vitamin D level:**
    A. Giant cell tumour
    B. Giant cell reparative granuloma
    C. Nonossifying fibroma
    D. Fibrous dysplasia
    E. Malignant fibrous histiocytoma

150. **Metastasis:**
    A. Carcinoma prostate produces hypocalcemia
    B. A cold spot is more common than hot spot in bone scan
    C. Prostate cancer is the most common cause of head less scan
    D. Anaplastic carcinomas produce hot spot
    E. Healing is usually marked by progressive decrease in uptake

151. **Aneurysmal bone cyst can arise secondary to:**
    A. Nonossifying fibroma
    B. Osteoblastoma
    C. Brown tumour
    D. Malignant fibrous histiocytoma
    E. Chondroblastoma

152. **Soft tissue complications of osteochondroma:**
    A. Bursitis
    B. Tenosynovitis
    C. Dysphagia
    D. Haematuria
    E. Soft tissue snapping

ANSWERS

1. **A-T, B-F, C-T, D-T, E-T**
   Cartilage containing tumours—enchondroma, chondroblastoma, CMF, chondrosarcoma
   Bone containing tumours—osteoblastoma, osteoid osteoma, osteosarcoma
   Fibrosarcoma, MFH

2. **A-T, B-T, C-T, D-T, E-F**
   Aneurysmal bone cyst is the most common before epiphyseal fusion and giant cell tumour after it. Degenerative geode, rheumatoid, gout, CPPD, hemophilia, chondroblastoma, benign fibrous histiocytoma, ganglion and metastases are other causes.

3. **A-T, B-T, C-T, D-T, E-F**
   Telangiectactic osteosarcoma, plasmacytoma, enchondroma and conventional chondrosarcoma produce expansion. Other lesions are metastasis from thyroid, kidney, pheochromocytoma, melanoma, breast, lung. Aneurysmal bone cyst and giant cell tumour are most common causes.

4. **A-T, B-T, C-T, D-F, E-T**
   Nonossifying fibroma and aneurysmal bone cyst are other causes.

5. **A-T, B-T, C-T, D-T, E-T**
   Metastasis, osteosarcoma, lymphoma, chondrosarcoma and MFH are other causes.

6. **A-T, B-T, C-T, D-T, E-F**
   Enchondroma, eosinophilic granuloma are other causes.

7. **A-F, B-T, C-T, D-F, E-T**
   Osteosarcoma 2-3 decade, parosteal 3-4 : SBC 1-2.

8. **A-T, B-F, C-T, D-T, E-F**
   Osteoma 3-5 decade. Hemangioma 3-7 decade.

9. **A-T, B-T, C-T, D-T, E-F**
   Osteosarcoma has a double peak, 1-2 decade and 7th decade
   Lymphoma also has a double peak. Fibrosarcoma and MFH are common in the 3-4 decades.

10. **A-F, B-T, C-T, D-T, E-T**
    Ewing's, metastasis, lymphoma, myeloma and chondrosarcoma are other diaphyseal tumours.

11. **A-T, B-F, C-F, D-T, E-T**
    Peripheral chondrosarcoma arises here. Chondroblastoma and benign fibrous histiocytoma are in epiphysis. Osteosarcoma, simple

bone cyst, osteoblastoma, nonossifying fibroma are other meta-physeal.

12. **A-T, B-T, C-T, D-T, E-T**
   Ewing's, osteosarcoma, eosinophilic granuloma, metastasis, fibrosarcoma and MFH are other causes.

13. **A-T, B-T, C-T, D-F, E-T**
   Benign osteogenic tumour, common in vertebra than in peripheral skeleton. In periphery, it is seen predominantly in diaphysis. 2,3 decade, males. There are aggressive variants, which recur frequently. Can be differentiated only pathologically.

14. **A-T, B-T, C-F, D-F, E-T**
   By definition, osteoblastoma has a nidus large than 1.5 cm, osteoid osteoma less than 1.5 cm. Produces severe pain, but relief with salicylates is not as common as in osteoid osteoma. In spine, it is common in the posterior elements.

15. **A-T, B-T, C-T, D-T, E-T**
   Simple bone cyst, enchondroma, chondroblastoma and geode are other causes.

16. **A-T, B-T, C-T, D-T, E-F**
   Soft tissue component can be seen.

17. **A-T, B-F, C-T, D-T, E-T**
   Pathologically, it is the same as osteoblastoma and only the size can differentiate them. There is a osteoid nidus with vascular connective tissue and reactive sclerosis. Nocturnal pain, relieved by salicylates.

18. **A-T, B-T, C-T, D-T, E-T**
   Typical appearance is a diaphyseal lucency with rim of sclerosis, with laminated periosteal reaction. No soft tissue component.

19. **A-T, B-T, C-F, D-F, E-F**
   One of the few bone tumours to metastasise to bone. Head and neck has best prognosis. Periosteal reaction is seen in early stage before appearance of lysis in bone. The bone grows longitudinal instead of concentric pattern, involving the whole shaft.

20. **A-T, B-T, C-F, D-F, E-T**
   Bone scan shows double density, increased uptake in the center and more intense uptake peripherally. MRI shows nidus isointense in T1 and low in T2.

21. **A-F, B-F, C-T, D-T, E-T**
It is seen in Gardner's syndrome, in which there are colonic polyps and osteomas. It is common in the outer table of skull and in the paranasal sinuses, frontal being the most common.

22. **A-F, B-T, C-T, D-T, E-F**
Seen in children less than five years. Majority in tibia. 20% have associated fibular involvement. Expansile lesion with sclerotic rim, with thinning of cortex, similar to fibrous dysplasia. Many undergo spontaneous regression.

23. **A-F, B-F, C-F, D-F, E-F**
Presents after epiphyseal closure, 20-40 years being peak age. It is eccentric, subarticular, expansile, multilocular, cortical destruction and soft tissue seen. Most common in distal femur. Periosteal reaction seen only if there is pathological fractures.

24. **A-F, B-T, C-T, D-T, E-F**
It arises from notochordal remnants. Common in the sacral and spheno-occipital region.
Pathologically there are physaliphorous cells with low mitotic activity. It is a malignant tumour with very slow growth.

25. **A-F, B-T, C-T, D-F, E-T**
Characteristic findings are well-defined bone destruction, with large soft tissue component, which may occasionally calcify. The soft tissue component extends anteriorly and can cause bladder and rectal compression. Equal sex incidence before 40 years.

26. **A-F, B-F, C-F, D-T, E-F**
It is usually a non-Hodgkin's lymphoma and majority are high-grade large cell lymphomas. It usually affects the diaphysis of long bones, but flat bones are also affected. Seen in 20 and 50 years.

27. **A-T, B-F, C-T, D-T, E-T**
Reactive sclerosis is a characteristic feature, seen in more than 50% of X-rays. Moth-eaten or permeative pattern seen. Seen predominantly in long bones. Presence of lung metastasis also excludes primary lymphoma.

28. **A-F, B-T, C-F, D-T, E-T**
Most common malignant tumour in children. Usually medullary origin. But can orginate from subperiosteal region. Can present with an infective picture. Common age group is 5-15 years.

29. **A-T, B-T, C-T, D-F, E-F**
Soft tissue mass is well-defined unlike osteomyelitis where it is ill-defined. Flat bone tumours produce reactive sclerosis making

it difficult to distinguish from osteosarcoma. Sunburst spiculation is sparse. Dynamic MRI is useful for assessing response to chemotherapy. Lung metastasis is the most common.

30. **A-T, B-T, C-T, D-T, E-T**
Osteomyelitis—same clinical features. Periosteal reaction earliest finding. Ill-defined soft tissue mass with disrupted soft tissue planes.
Neuroblastoma—younger age group, multiple, metaphyseal
Eosinophilic granuloma—solid periosteal reaction
Osteosarcoma—sclerosis, ossification, solid dense sunburst periosteal reaction.
Lymphoma—older age group, systemic symptoms less common, has similar appearance with sclerosis and diaphyseal involvement with same pathological appearances.

31. **A-T, B-F, C-F, D-F, E-T**
Nidus is usually lucent, but it can be calcified or completely sclerotic. Scoliosis is painful and concave to the same side of the lesion. There is no sclerosis if the lesion is subperiosteal.

32. **A-F, B-T, C-T, D-F, E-T**
Intra-articular lesions are difficult to detect. There is little or no sclerosis. Premature osteoarthritis seen.
Joint space is increased due to reactive effusion or synovitis.

33. **A-T, B-F, C-F, D-T, E-F**
Eosinophilic granuloma is the most common presentation of histiocytosis. A well-defined lucent lesion with sclerosis, endosteal scalloping, occasionally expansile and periosteal reaction can be multiloculated. In skull, multiple punched out lesions with bevelled edge, geographical skull; vertebra plana, floating teeth are presentations.

34. **A-T, B-T, C-F, D-T, E-T**
Metastasis, tuberculosis, chondrosarcoma, GCT are others.

35. **A-F, B-T, C-T, D-T, E-T**
It commonly affects the angle of the mandible, more common in the mandible and males. The main histological types are follicular and plexiform types. The most common appearance is multilocular type with expansion of bone and floating teeth.

36. **A-F, B-T, C-T, D-T, E-F**
Chondroma, osteomyelitis, histiocytosis X, hemangioma, ABC, mets, myeloma, chondrosarcoma, osteosarcoma, lymphoma, Ewing's sarcoma.

37. **A-T, B-T, C-T, D-T, E-T**

   All these tumours have round cells in the pathological specimen.

38. **A-T, B-T, C-T, D-F, E-F**

   Neuroblastoma is the most common tumour with increased uptake in the bone scan.

39. **A-F, B-T, C-T, D-T, E-T**

   Associated with POEMS syndrome, which has polyneuropathy, organomegaly, endocrinopathy, multiple myeloma. Bone scan usually shows cold spot. There might be a hot rim around cold spot, called doughnut sign. Normal bone scan with uptake in gallium scan indicates rapid progressive disease. Increased uptake in bone scan is seen in pathological fracture or amyloid. Myeloma is hypointense in T1 and hyper in T2. After treatment, it becomes hypointense in both sequences.

40. **A-T, B-F, C-F, D-F, E-F**

   Myeloma, lymphoma and metastasis are the common lesions which cross the joint and involve multiple surfaces. Sclerosis is seen in only 1.5% of cases. It can be spontaneous or may be due to chemotherapy or radiotherapy or fractures. Extramedullary plasmacytoma occurs in younger population and has a 30% conversion to multiple myeloma which is lesser than that for solitary plasmacytoma. Alkaline phosphatase is normal in multiple myeloma, unlike osteoporosis circumscripta which is Paget's disease in skull, with high alkaline phosphatase.

41. **A-F, B-T, C-F, D-T, E-T**

   Feature of myeloma—diffuse osteoporosis with lytic focus in bodies, multiple vertebrae, extension to disc and contiguous vertebrae, pedicle sign is usually negative and late, anterior scalloping is common, soft tissue and pathological fracture are common. Osteolytic type is more common than sclerotic, diffuse osteosclerosis is rare and are symmetrical. Metastasis—lytic lesion in pedicle, pedicle sign positive and early, usually single vertebra, does not cross disc, anterior scalloping less common, soft tissue and pathological fracture rare, can be lytic or osteosclerotic, diffuse osteosclerosis can be seen, asymmetric. Alkaline phosphatase and phosphorus are normal, hypercalcemia is seen, unlike Paget's, in which there is elevated alkaline phosphatase, with normal calcium and phosphorus.

42. **A-T, B-T, C-F, D-T, E-T**

   The tumour grows in the subperiosteal region producing erosion of outer cortex. Onion peel pattern is seen in Ewing's, but is not specific. Due to periods of growth. The tumour arises centrally but migrates to eccentric location.

43. **A-F, B-T, C-T, D-T, E-T**
Bone scan generally overestimates the extent of osteosarcoma due to diffuse uptake. CT should be done before chemotherapy or surgery for excluding lung metastasis.

44. **A-T, B-T, C-F, D-F, E-F**
It happens in 3-4 decades. The mandibular lesions are lytic, with extensive periosteal reaction. Maxillary lesions are sclerotic.

45. **A-T, B-T, C-F, D-F, E-F**
This is a very aggressive, expansile tumour with haemorrhage and necrosis. Same age group, same bones, metaphyseal. Expansile lesion, geographical pattern, no sclerosis, may have ossification. Doughnut sign, central cold and peripheral high uptake.

46. **A-T, B-T, C-T, D-T, E-F**
Myositis ossificans—post-traumatic, calcification from periphery to center, clear demarcation from bone. CT finds extent of tumour in the intramedullary and soft tissue spaces MRI is better for assessing the intramedullary extension.

47. **A-F, B-T, C-T, D-T, E-F**
Multiple myeloma is the most common primary malignant bone tumour followed by OS.
Peak age is 20-30 years. Older age tumours can be due to Paget's, or irradiation or in jaw or independent of these factors. Majority are of osteoblastic pathology.

48. **A-F, B-T, C-T, D-T, E-F**
It usually affects metaphysis. Growth plate only delays spread to epiphysis. Tumours are very large at presentation. One of the few tumours to metastasise to lymph nodes. In early stages no bony changes are seen. Only periosteal reaction is seen. Bony destruction is a permeative pattern which is more aggressive than moth-eaten pattern.

49. **A-F, B-T, C-T, D-T, E-T**
Sunburst periosteal reaction is perpendicular to the cortex and also seen in Ewing's. Codman's triangle is also seen in other malignancies such as Ewing's and osteomyelitis. Soft tissue extension is very essential for prognosis and management.

50. **A-T, B-T, C-T, D-F, E-F**
Seen in 30-40 years age group. Less vascular.

51. **A-F, B-T, C-T, D-F, E-F**

Common in fourth and fifth decades. Femur is the most common long bone involved. Innominate bone is the most common flat bone. Pathological fractures are seen in 17%.

52. **A-T, B-T, C-T, D-T, E-T**

Most common second tumour in retinoblastoma. Metallic implants are also associated.

53. **A-F, B-T, C-F, D-T, E-T**

Majority are osteosarcoma followed by fibrosarcoma and MFH. It is also seen in monostotic disease. Any bone involved by Paget's can be affected. Usually spine is spared. Bone scans are not very useful. But a focal cold spot in a known Paget's is suggestive.

54. **A-T, B-F, C-T, D-F, E-T**

Chondroblastoma is seen in epiphyseal region, NOF is diametaphyseal, becoming metaphyseal.

55. **A-F, B-T, C-F, D-T, E-T**

Mandible is affected more commonly in myeloma than metastasis. Extrapleural masses are also seen in metastasis of primary bone tumours.

56. **A-F, B-T, C-T, D-F, E-T**

Adamantinoma is a malignant tumour, in tibial diaphysis, 10-50 years, males, lytic, central/eccentric, well-defined margin, sclerosis not seen, multiloculation and satellite lesions seen. Locally aggressive. Metastasis to lung.

57. **A-F, B-T, C-T, D-F, E-T**

The types of chondrosarcomas are conventional intramedullary, dedifferentiated, myxoid, mesenchymal, clear cell, telangiectatic and extraskeletal. Clear cell tumours are low-grade. Dedifferentiated tumours are characterised by dedifferentiation of low-grade tumours into high-grade sarcomatous elements. This is called collision of two tumours. Myxoid tumours are more common in soft tissue.

58. **A-T, B-T, C-T, D-T, E-F**

Rings and arcs of calcification is specific pattern for chondrogenic tumours. Lobular architecture is specific for hyaline cartilage containing tumours. Although chondrosarcoma is a malignant tumour, it is a slow growing tumour and it causes endosteal scalloping of bone when it tries to expand and break through compartments. More than 50% of tumours are larger than 10 cm. The tumour destroys the cortex and extends to soft tissue.

59. **A-F, B-T, C-T, D-F, E-F**
It arises sporadically or from juxtacortical osteochondroma. These tumours are of low-grade. They have a pseudocapsule and they do not invade the medulla. They can cause cortical erosion.

60. **A-T, B-F, C-F, D-F, E-F**
Rings of arcs or flocculent calcification is seen. Higher grade tumours have less calcification. Permeative pattern is seen in high-grade tumours such as mesenchymal and dedifferentiated tumours. The depth of endosteal scalloping is more important than the length of scalloping. If the scalloping is .> 2/3rd of cortical thickness, it is likely to be malignant, rather than enchondroma. Soft tissue extension occurs in chondrosarcomas.

61. **A-T, B-T, C-T, D-T, E-T**

62. **A-T, B-F, C-T, D-F, E-T**
Parosteal osteosarcoma—3rd, 4th decade; Males = Females, metaphysis of distal femur, tibia; Dense mass of bone surrounding shaft; sattelite lesions seen, initially a lucencey separates tumor from cortex, later involves cortex and medulla.

63. **A-T, B-T, C-T, D-T, E-F**
The density of the lesion is low due to hyaline cartilage. Septal enhancement and rim enhancement is more common in low-grade tumours. High-grade tumours show diffuse or nodular enhancement.

64. **A-T, B-T, C-T, D-T, E-T**

65. **A-T, B-F, C-T, D-F, E-F**
Chondroma—younger age, diaphyseal, hair on end periosteal reaction, osteoblastic component.

66. **A-T, B-T, C-T, D-F, E-F**
The lesion is usually high signal in T2 and low signal in T1. High signal in T1 may be seen due to entrapment of fatty marrow. Low signal in T2 is seen in high-grade tumour.
MRI is very useful for assessing soft tissue and bone marrow extension. Dynamic MRI is not very useful for assessing grade.

67. **A-T, B-F, C-T, D-T, E-T**
In ribs chondrosarcomas are more common than enchondromas. They are seen in anterior aspect of ribs and are common in a younger age. In short bones, enchondromas are more common than chondrosarcomas and they are associated with prominent endosteal scalloping. Enchondromas are rare in pelvic bones, but it is the most common flat bone site of chondrosarcomas, majority arising close to triradiate cartilage.

68. **A-F, B-F, C-T, D-F, E-F**
    It is commonly seen in femur and in the epiphysis. It constitutes
    1-2% of chondrosarcomas. It is lower grade than conventional
    chondrosarcomas and has a better prognosis than it.

69. **A-T, B-F, C-T, D-T, E-F**
    Nonossifying fibromas are benign lesions made up of whorled
    fibroblasts, in the bony cortex, common in males,(2:1), and less
    than 20 years. These are called fibrous cortical defects if less than
    2 cm and nonossifying fibroma, when more than 2 cm. These
    lesions are seen in 50% of asymptomatic boys and 20% of
    asymptomatic girls. They are common in tibia and femur. They
    are situated eccentrically in the cortex (posterior and medial
    cortices common) in the metaphyseal and metadiaphyseal region.
    They may grow into diaphysis when they are large. They are well-
    defined lytic lesions with sclerotic or serpentine margins. Larger
    lesions are expansile and multiloculated.

70. **A-T, B-T, C-F, D-T, E-T**
    Pathologic fractures are uncommon in nonossifying fibroma. Soft
    tissue mass or periostitis suggests an aggressive lesion and should
    be further investigated. Multiple ossifying fibromas when
    associated with extraskeletal abnormalities like mental retardation,
    ocular abnormalities, café au lait spots, hypogonadism and
    cryptorchidism, is called Jaffe-Campanacci syndrome. The non-
    ossifying fibromas eventually become sclerotic due to fibro-osseous
    proliferation. Occasionally, they may enlarge, or become smaller
    or disappear completely.

71. **A-T, B-T, C-F, D-T, E-T**
    It is a low-grade tumour. Hence there is a rind of sclerosis. Soft
    tissue component is uncommon.
    T2 is heterogeneous

72. **A-T, B-T, C-T, D-T, E-T**
    Uptake is seen in bone scan and DMSA, which is not seen in
    enchondroma. Soft tissue is also more common in chondrosarcoma
    than enchondroma.

73. **A-F, B-T, C-T, D-T, E-T**
    I—synchronous, < five months, <18 yrs
    II—synchronous, < 5 months, > 18 yrs
    IIIa—metachronous, 5-24 months
    IIIb—metachronous, 24 months
    In late stages, the bone is completely sclerotic. Metastasis is seen,
    metaphyseal.

74. **A-T, B-F, C-F, D-T, E-T**
Intermediate grade tumour with better prognosis. The tumour is attached to the cortex, which is thickened and scalloped. Periosteal reaction and soft tissue seen. No cortical destruction.

75. **A-F, B-T, C-T, D-T, E-F**
Chondrosarcomas are high signal in T2W images, whereas chondroblastomas are low to intermediate signal intensity. Periosteal reaction is more common than in enchondromas, which do not have it, unless there is fracture.

76. **A-F, B-F, C-F, D-F, E-F**
Medullary cavity is not involved. The cortex is thickened.
Seen in 3rd-4th decade. Very rare in innominate bone. It is common in posterior aspect of distal femoral metaphysis.

77. **A-T, B-F, C-T, D-T, E-T**
The tumours can be low-grade, but eventually get converted into high-grade tumour. There are many theories for this conversion. 1) malignant transformation of low-grade tumour, 2) malignant conversion of pseudocapsule of low-grade tumour, and 3) simultaneous origin of low and high-grade tumour. In CT—low-grade is hypodense, high-grade is isodense. In MRI low-grade, Hypo in T1, hyper in T2, peripheral or septal enhancement.
High-grade—hypo to intermediate in T1, T2, diffuse, nodular enhancement.

78. **A-F, B-T, C-T, D-F, E-T**
Arises from synovial lining of bursa or tendon sheaths. It is usually seen in males, 30-50 years age.

79. **A-F, B-T, C-T, D-T, E-T**
Ossifying fibromas is a benign tumour which has pathological and radiological similarities to fibrous dysplasia. It has a well-vascularised fibrous stroma with trabeculae of new bone, rimmed by osteoblasts. The osteoblastic rimming is the main pathological feature differentiating it from fibrous dysplasia. It is seen in diaphysis, unlike metaphysical location of FD. It occurs one decade earlier than FD, at 1st and 2nd decade. It is seen in facial bones, common in females.Affects tibia more common than fibula. It can involve entire circumference of fibula. It starts in the cortex, extends to the medulla, can be lytic sclerotic or ground glass, with band of sclerosis. Can be uni or multilocular, with pathological fracture and pseudoarthrosis.

80. **A-T, B-T, C-T, D-T, E-T**
Nonossifying fibroma is the most common tumour with this appearance. This is eccentric, well-defined, lucent, metaphysic

Osteoid osteoma—cortical lucency, sclerosis, thickening
Brodie's abscess—thick rim of sclerosis.
Chondromyxoid fibroma—trabeculated, extends to diaphysis or epiphysis.
Focal fibrocartilaginous dysplasia—medial aspect of proximal tibia
Herniation pit—lucent lesion in lateral aspect of femoral neck
Periosteal desmoid—saucer-like defect, with sclerosis and periostitis.

81. A-F, B-T, C-F, D-T, E-F

There is no communication with the joint. It is caused due to intraosseous mucoid degeneration.

The lesion is well-defined, lytic with a rim of sclerosis. There is increased uptake in 10%. In MRI, the lesion is isointense in T1 and hyperintense in T2, but no internal septations are seen like in the soft tissue ganglion. Seen in epiphysis, subchondral portion.

82. A-T, B-T, C-T, D-T, E-F, F-F

Epiphyseal extension is vey rare. The dorsal spine is involved more than lumbar, cervical vertebrae. The tumours typically arise eccentrically from the bone. But occasionally they can arise from the centre of the bone, especially in fibula. The incidence of secondary ABC varies from 1-30%. The tumour has cavernous spaces lined by fibrous tissue without endothelial lining.

83. A-T, B-T, C-F, D-F, E-F

Healing of pathological fracture depends on the location and the primary tumour. Bone is usually involved by hematogenous spread which can be arterial or venous. Lymphatic spread is rare because bone has no lymphatics, but the primary tumour can spread to the lymph nodes which then secondarily involve the adjacent bones. Medulloblastoma is the most common brain tumour to spread by CSF, followed by ependymoma, pineal tumours, astrocytomas and lymphoma. In prostate cancer, the metastasis spreads through the Batson's plexus of veins. Hence bones are involved before lung.

84. A-T, B-T, C-T, D-F, E-F

The lesion can show many variants. Can be completely solid or completely intracortical. Injection of ethibloc should be done careful as it can cause inflammation of spinal cord and nerve roots. The entire lesion is predominantly hypovascular, but can show patchy hypervascular areas. It can occasionally extend into soft tissue.

85. **A-T, B-F, C-T, D-F, E-F**
Malignant—osteosarcoma, Ewing's sarcoma, neuroblastoma metastasis; Benign—histiocytosis, fibrous cortical defect, aneurysmal bone cyst, nonossifying fibroma, chondroblastoma.

86. **A-F, B-T, C-T, D-F, E-T**
Osteomas project from the surface of the bone and there is no communication with the medullary cavity of the parent bone. Bone infarctions are seen in the medulla, are lucent with peripheral shell of calcification. Bone island is also seen in the medulla, round or oblong, has thorny radiating spicules. Ostoid ·osteoma can be seen in the cortex, medulla or subperiosteal region. The most common are in the cortex, where there is lucency surrounded by calcification and sclerosis. Medullary osteroid osteomas are lucent or calcified, but there is no sclerosis. Subperiosteal lesions are scalloped with calcification. Sclerosis is seen.

87. **A-F, B-T, C-T, D-F, E-F**
20-30 years. Tibia> femur> ribs. Located in metaphysic. Well-defined lytic with sclerotic rim. Septations are seen. Calcification can be seen, but it is not common.

88. **A-F, B-T, C-F, D-T, E-F**
Lumbar vertebra is the most common involved followed by dorsal vertebra. The disk height is preserved unlike infection. Breast metastasis has a high incidence in L2 and lung metastasis in D12. Destruction of the vertebra, soft tissue, fracture, and spinal cord compression by extradural or intradural mass.

89. **A-F, B-T, C-T, D-T, E-F**
Carcinoid metastasis are sclerotic. Renal metastatis are lytic and expansile.

90. **A-T, B-T, C-F, D-F, E-T**
Thyroid, kidney, adrenal, uterus, Wilms, Ewing's, pheochromcytoma, melanoma, hepatoma, SC skin, vascular tumours and soft tissue sarcoma.

91. **A-T, B-F, C-T, D-F, E-F**
Prostate, carcinoid, bladder, nasopharynx, stomach, medulloblastoma and neuroblastoma are sclerotic. Ovarian, lung, breast, cervix and testicular tumours are mixed.

92. **A-T, B-T, C-T, D-T, E-F**
This is a high-grade tumour, which is common in the axial skeleton, especially in maxilla and mandible. It constitutes 2-13% of chondrosarcomas and seen in 2-4th decade.

The tumour has a permeative pattern with soft tissue component. There is fine stippled calcificaiton. MRI—intermediate signal due to low water content. Serpentine vessels are seen inside the lesion suggesting high-grade vascular tumour. Contrast enhancement is more of delayed intense enhancement. Enhancement is diffuse. No peripheral or septal enhancement is seen.

93. A-T, B-T, C-F, D-F, E-F
Periosteal reaction, soft tissue mass in both.

94. A-F, B-T, C-T, D-F, E-F
Batson's plexus is an intercommunicating system of thin-walled veins surrounding the spinal column. They do not have valves. The flow is slow and is variable in any direction. It is not subject to direct pressure of thoracoabdominal muscles, but varies with coughing, sneezing and straining. The veins communicate with veins in spinal canal, caval, portal, azygos, intercostal, pulmonary, and renal veins.

95. A-F, B-F, C-T, D-T, E-F
Stromal bone formation is due to intramembranous ossification of fibrous stroma and is seen in carcinoma prostate. Reactive bone formation is reactive response to bone destruction and this is immature bone. This is seen in leukemia, lymphoma and plasmacytoma. Medullary lesions are detected later, because of fewer trabeculae and endosteal erosion can be the earliest sign. Lung, colon, kidney and uterus are the most common tumours to spread to legs by retrograde venous spread. Involvement below elbows and knees are uncommon because of paucity of red marrow. Bronchogenic cancer is the most common to metastasise at these locations.

96. A-F, B-F, C-T, D-F, E-T
In metastasis, hypercalcemia is produced due to bone resorption, immobilisation and release of PTH. Alkaline phosphatase is elevated in bone metastasis independent of liver involvement. An osteolytic lesion heals by becoming smaller and ossifying progressively from periphery to center and becoming completely sclerotic. Mixed lesions usually become smaller and sclerotic. Sclerotic lesions, if healing, become smaller and may disappear completely. Appearance of a new sclerotic lesion after treatment can indicate a new metastasis, but it may also indicate healing of a subradiological small lytic metastasis.

97. A-T, B-T, C-T, D-T, E-F
GIT tumours are other common causes. It is common in blastic lesions and common in lower extremities.

98. **A-F, B-F, C-F, D-T, E-F**
    Hypercalcemia, bone pain, normocytic normochromic anemia are common features. Bence Jones proteinuria is seen only in 50%. Monoclonal protein production. Majority are in 50-80 years age group. Stippling is seen in lead poisoning.

99. **A-T, B-T, C-T, D-F, E-T**
    Myeloma is cold or normal in bone scan. It usually underestimates the extent. Sclerosis is usually seen following radiation, but there are purely sclerotic tumours. Periosteal reaction is uncommon even if there is infarction.

100. **A-T, B-F, C-T, D-F, E-T**
     Majority of the metastasis are multiple. Moth-eaten pattern of destruction is most common in breast cancer. Soft tissue calcification is often seen in colonic cancer metastasis. Soft tissue involvement is more common in rib metastasis than in other places. Pathological fracture is more common in vertebra than proximal femur.

101. **A-T, B-T, C-T, D-T, E-F**
     Osteochondromas comprise 35% of all benign bone tumours. 65% are situated around knee and proximal humerus, 20% occur in axial skeleton and 5% occur in the spine. Arise in metaphysis or metadiaphyseal region. Epiphyseal origin is rare.

102. **A-F, B-T, C-T, D-T, E-T**
     Grow away from the joint. Growth usually parallels the host bone, but occasionally may overgrow the skeletal maturity. Complications are directly related to size and site. The actively growing portion is the cartilage cap.

103. **A-F, B-T, C-T, D-T, E-F**
     Chronic renal failure is more common than acute renal failure. Non-ionic contrast should be given and hydration should be adequate. Amyloidosis seen in 20%. ESR elevated due to proteins. Waldenström's macroglobulinemia produces similar radiological appearances. IgM raised in Waldenströms.

104. **A-T, B-T, C-F, D-T, E-T**
     X-rays have 90% sensitivity, as compared to bone with 75% sensitivity. In head, there are multiple punched out lesions, with mandibular involvement unlike mets.

105. **A-T, B-T, C-F, D-T, E-T**
     50-75% are solitary. Seen in children, usually 4-7 years. Long bones, skull, pelvis, flat bones affected, 20% multiple.

106. **A-F, B-T, C-F, D-T, E-T**

Associated with diabetes insipidus, not mellitus. More common in men than women. In the lungs, there are nodules initially, followed by cysts and subsequently fibrosis and end stage lung. Hand-Schüller disease has diabetes insipidus, exophthalmos, pulmonary disease, skin lesions, lymph nodes, hepatosplenomegaly.

107. **A-T, B-T, C-T, D-T, E-T**

Bone scan is usually photophrenic, but can show increased uptake. Polka dot appearance is due to thickened trabeculae in cross section.

108. **A-T, B-T, C-T, D-F, E-T**

Coarse trabeculae in cross section gives Polka dot appearance.

109. **A-T, B-F, C-F, D-T, E-F**

The signal in hemangiomas depend on the amount of fat and the rate of blood flow.

If there is low flow, the lesion is low in T1, high in T2. If there is high flow, the lesion is low in all sequence. In vertebral hemangiomas because of the fat, the lesion can be high in both sequences. Majority of osseous hemangiomas are cavernous, but vertebral are usually capillary with fat in them. More the fat, less the symptoms for the patient.

110. **A-T, B-T, C-T, D-F, E-T**

Bone island and fibrous dysplasias are other tumours which are known to regress spontaneously.

111. **A-F, B-T, C-T, D-F, E-T**

Paget's—Osteosarcoma > fibrosarcoma > malignant fibrous histiocytoma.

112. **A-T, B-T, C-T, D-F, E-T**

Chronic friction results in the development of a bursa between the cartilage cap and adjacent muscles and tendons. This is hypo in T1 and hyper in T2 weighted images and shows rim enhancement. The inflamed bursa makes early diagnosis possible and the presence of bursa usually indicates a benign process.

113. **A-T, B-T, C-T, D-T, E-T**

Soft tissue hemangiomas are usually cavernous or capillary. They have a large fatty component. The MRI signal is variable. It can be hyperintense in both T1 and T2 due to fat or haemorrhage. Serpentine flow voids are seen. Synovial hemangioma is seen due to repeated joint haemorrhages.

114. **A-F, B-F, C-T, D-T, E-T**
Pseudoaneurysm is common in the distal superficial femoral artery (trapped between the adductor hiatus and geniculate branches) and popliteal artery. Sessile osteochondromas are more prone for causing pseudoaneurysm due to chronic pressure, rather than pedunculated lesions which just displace. Common peroneal nerve is the commonly affected nerve and it is diagnosed by atrophic changes in short head of biceps femoris and extensor muscles of leg.

115. **A-T, B-T, C-T, D-F, E-T**
Positive metacarpal sign—In a normal person, a line drawn tangential to the head of the fourth and fifth metacarpal, does not intersect the 3rd metacarpal bone or just touches the head. If the line intersects the 3rd metacarpal, it is positive metacarpal sign and indicates a short 4th and 5th metacarpal. The common cause of this sign is hypoparathyroidism and pseudohypothyroidism. Other causes include Turner's syndrome, Beckwith-Wiedemann syndrome and basal cell nevus syndrome.

116. **A-T, B-T, C-T, D-T, E-T**
Radial head subluxation is also common.

117. **A-T, B-F, C-T, D-T, E-T**
Risk of malignancy in osteochondroma—1% and 1-25% in diaphyseal aclasia. 90% are chondrosarcomas. Osteosarcoma, fibrosarcoma and spindle cell sarcoma comprise the other 10%. Chondrosarcomas are more common in the axial skeleton, the majority occurring in the pelvis, proximal femur and shoulder girdle.

118. **A-T, B-F, C-F, D-T, E-T**
Clinical—recent onset of unexplained pain, progressive growth
Radiological—cartilage cap > 2 cm, irregular surface, lucency within cartilage, soft tissue mass, scattered calcific foci, and destruction of adjacent bones.

119. **A-F, B-F, C-F, D-F, E-T**
Most common in the proximal humerus, proximal femur and iliac bone. Unilocular in more than 90% of cases. Recurrence is more in younger children and in lesions abuting growth plate in the epiphysis. Normally, these are seen in metaphysis.

120. **A-F, B-T, C-T, D-F, E-T**
The lesion is centrally placed in the cortex, expansile with a rim of sclerosis. Mild expansion, cortical thinning and pathological fractures are common. Lesions in diaphysis are larger, have well-

defined sclerosis and is inactive. In calcaneum the lesion is seen anteriorly. It has a straight border anteriorly and curvilinear posterior border which is parallel to the posterior trabeculae.

121. A-T, B-T, C-T, D-T, E-T
Hemothorax is usually secondary to rib exostosis.

122. A-T, B-T, C-T, D-T, E-T
The falling fragment sign refers to a vertical fracture fragment, which moves within the cyst. Percutaneous treatments. include injection of MPA (Medroxyprogesterone acetate), which produces complete healing in 90%. The mechanism of action is believed to be a reparative response to injection or direct effect on the cellular component. If there is recurrence, ethibloc is used. This arrests the further growth of tumour, induces osteosclerosis and strengthens the bone. Autologous bone marrow can also be injected.

123. A-T, B-T, C-T, D-T, E-T
Giant cell tumour, giant cell reparating granuloma, nonossifying fibroma, brown tumour, simple bone cyst, chondroblastoma and ossifying fibroma are other tumours with giant cell.

124. A-T, B-T, C-T, D-T, E-F
Giant cell tumour and aneurysmal bone cyst are the common tumours with multiple septations, giving a soap bubble appearance.

125. A-T, B-T, C-F, D-T, E-T
40% of lesions are lytic with multiple septations. The septations can be sparse, thin or modest thick or coarse and indistinct. The lesions are seen in the subchondral region, eccentric, expansile with cortical thinning. In the calcaneum, it occurs in the posterior aspect unlike simple bone cyst which occurs anteriorly. Lesions in the ilium are purely lytic without trabeculations. Lesions in sternum, vertebrae and ribs have a lot of soft tissue. For three months after treatment, the lesion increases clinically and radiologically. After this, the lesion gradually recalcifies and heals.

126. A-F, B-T, C-T, D-T, E-T
Radiation-induced sarcomas diagnostic criteria 1. radiation, 2. tumour developing in radiation field, 3. significant latent period (3-4 years), and 4. histologic confirmation. Osteosarcomas are the most common radiation-induced sarcomas, even though the primary is extraosseous. Malignant fibrous histiocytomas are the most common soft tissue sarcomas. The latent period is longer for the bone sarcomas. Bimodal age distribution is seen in soft tissue sarcomas.

127. **A-T, B-T, C-T, D-T, E-T**

The common treatments of giant cell tumour include radiation, curettage and bone grafting and surgery. All the benign recurrences occur within four years. Any recurrence after five years is suspicious of malignancy. GCT in Paget's will be seen as areas of lucency within Paget's bone. Giant cell tumour has the peculiar feature of being transported in the bloodstream and implanted in distal sites. These are not metastasis and do not worsen prognosis. This is also seen in chondroblastoma and is common in the distal radial tumours.

128. **A-T, B-T, C-T, D-T, E-T**

A histologically benign tumour can metastasise. This is different from distal implantation. Malignant GCTs can be primarily malignant or a conversion of benign GCT. They have bad prognosis. Seeding in soft tissue during surgery gives soft tissue tumour. Chondrosarcomas and osteosarcomas are more common after radiation than giant cell tumour.

129. **A-F, B-F, C-F, D-F, E-T**

Doses higher than 10 Gy are carcinogenic. Higher doses > 50 Gy cause complete cell death and there is no significant risk for cancer, whereas doses 30-50 Gy cause only partial damage and mutations and affect reparative mechanisms, resulting in second cancers. The risk is higher in the periphery of field, which receives lesser in homogeneous dose. Prognosis is limited by surgical resectability. The trunk and limb girdle lesions have worse prognosis than the craniofacial lesions. Chemotherapy increases the risk.

130. **A-T, B-T, C-F, D-T, E-T**

MRI is very sensitive. Fatty hyperintensity is seen in postradiation T1 films and development of soft tissue is an earlier finding. Soft tissue mass, bone destruction, osteoid or chondroid mineralisation and periosteal reaction, in a patient whose X-rays were stable for five years, point towards the diagnosis. Isolated periosteal reaction is nonspecific and may be secondary to fracture.

131. **A-T, B-T, C-F, D-F, E-F**

All multiple chondromas are not necessarily Ollier's. Ollier's have wide distribution, unilateral, asymmetrical, multiple, deformed, shortened bones. X-ray shows linear or columnar lucencies in metaphysis with calcification and erosions. 30% malignant conversion.

132. **A-F, B-T, C-F, D-T, E-T**

Lymphomas, osteoid osteomas are diaphyseal.

133. A-T, B-F, C-T, D-F, E-F
Upper end of tibia and lower end of femur are common locations 10-30 years is common age. Lesions are metaphyseal and may extend into epiphysis
Smooth scalloped endosteal margin. Calcification is uncommon

134. A-T, B-T, C-T, D-T, E-F
Fibrous tissue has low signal in T1 and T2. Chronic haemorrhage has dark signal in boht sequences. The edema in the intial post-operative period has high signal in T2 and low in T1, but this is feathery with ill-defined margins.

135. A-F, B-T, C-F, D-F, E-F
Giant cell tumours are seen in subarticular lesions of the epiphysis. They can occasionally extend to the metaphysis or diaphysis. Aneurysmal bone cyst occurs before epiphyseal fusion, but giant cell tumours occur after epiphyseal fusion. They can pass through the cartilage and involve the joint space and adjacent bone. Internal septa are not due to new bone, but due to trabecular remnants or reactive ridges or grooves on endosteal surface of cortex overlying lesion. Periosteal reaction and sclerosis are not common. Periosteal reaction is seen in 10% and signifies periosteal reaction.

136. A-T, B-F, C-F, D-F, E-F
Sensitive to cold and not heat. Well-defined lytic lesion is seen in the terminal phalanx due to pressure erosion. Well seen only in the vascular phase and not in the standard static phase. Hemangiopericytomas are also considered benign. Implantation dermoid is a differential

137. A-F, B-F, C-T, D-F, E-T
Benign tumour; can be locally aggressive and metastasis very rare males; 2nd decade; epiphysis extending to metaphysis, well-defined, lucent, expansile, sclerotic rim, calcification 10-60%; periosteal reaction—1/3rd, linear; no soft tissue; secondary ABC can arise.

138. A-F, B-T, C-F, D-F, E-T
In schwannoma the nerve runs eccentric in the peri/epineurium, unlike neurofibroma where it runs through the mass. There are many variants of malignant schwannoma like Triton tumour, melanotic schwannoma, epitheloid and glandular schwannoma. It is very common in the peripheral nerves. Uncommon in cranial nerve, V nerve being most common. It is notorious for recurrence.

139. A-T, B-F, C-F, D-F, E-T
Although schwannomas can be sporadic, 50% are associated with neurofibromatosis. These tumours occur at younger age group, are

more aggressive histologically, have more sarcomatous elements, multiple, metastasise and are difficult to resect.

140. **A-F, B-T, C-T, D-T, E-T**
Solitary neurofibromas and neurilemmomas are not associated with NF-1, but localised neurofibromas are seen in the syndrome. Neurilemmomas are made up of Schwann cells and neurofibromas have mixed cell population. A characteristic feature of neurogenic tumours in ultrasound, is the presence of echogenic capsule in ultrasound. Ganglioneuroblastoma is a tumour that arises from the ganglia cells and is common in the retroperitoneum and posterior mediastinum.

141. **A-T, B-T, C-T, D-T, E-F**
Blastic metastasis, like that seen in prostate carcinoma are less likely to fracture than lytic lesions. 100% of patients with metastasis more than 50% of cortical surface involvement will fracture. There is no direct correlation between the size of the lesion and the risk of fracture. The subtrochanteric region is a typical example. Regardless of the size, any involvement of this region is prone for fracture. Presence of pain is the common indicator for surgical fixation.

142. **A-T, B-T, C-T, D-T, E-T**
It is mainly due to Epstein-Barr virus infection.

143. **A-T, B-F, C-F, D-T, E-T**
Lung cancer is less likely to present with pathological fracture as the patients do not live long enough. Breast cancer and prostate cancer are the most common causes. The most common presentation of bone metastasis is pain. This is due to stretching of periosteum or stimulation of endosteal nerve endings.

144. **A-F, B-T, C-F, D-F, E-T**
Fibromatosis is a benign, locally aggressive tumour. It is seen in subcutaneous tissue, fascia, tendons, muscles and bones. Superficial lesions are less aggressive. The lesion is heterogeneous and has low signal in T1 and T2.

145. **A-T, B-T, C-T, D-T, E-T**
Metastasis to muscle is very uncommon and indicates very advanced disease. It is also seen in lung cancers.

146. **A-T, B-T, C-F, D-T, E-F**
Lactic acid produced by tumour is essential for formation of new vessels, but in skeletal muscle this lactic acid is cleared very quickly. The pH of the muscle is also not ideal for tumour growth.

147. **A-T, B-F, C-T, D-T, E-T**
Telangiectatic osteosarcoma and chondroblastoma are other causes of fluid-fluid level.

148. **A-F, B-T, C-F, D-T, E-T**
Hip joint is the most common joint involved in periarticular spread without intra-articular extension. Knee is the most common joint with intra-articular extension. Except psoas, pelvic muscles are the most common muscles involved in metastases. Breast and lung are more common than leukemia in involving the synovium. Metastasis do not involve the discs because they are avascular and the cartilage has inhibitors for metastatic spread. But discal narrowing can be caused by metastasis-induced degenerative change due to interference with diffusion of fluid from marrow to the disc. If degenerative changes are seen only focally, where there is metastasis, it is likely to be secondary to the metastasis. Very rarely, metastasis can spread through the gaps in end plate into the disc. Hematogenous spread is extremely rare and is more common in children and happens in the periphery of the disc. If there is pure hematogenous spread to disc, only the disc space is narrowed without involvement of the vertebral bodies.

149. **A-T, B-T, C-T, D-T, E-T**
These tumours produce oncogenic rickets. There is low calcium, low phosphate, high alkaline phosphatase and low vitamin D. Other tumours are vascular tumours and osteoblastoma.

150. **A-T, B-F, C-T, D-F, E-T**
Usually metastasis produce hypercalcemia due to bone resorption and other causes. In prostate cancer, there is hypocalcemia due to bone deposition. Hot spot is more common than cold spot. Hot spot indicates increased flow or increased turnover due to reactive bone deposition. Cold spot is due to complete resorption of bone. There is no reactive response in plasmacytoma, anaplastic carcinoma and leukemia. Healing usually is marked by progressive fall in uptake, while progress shows increased uptake. A rapidly enlarging lytic lesion becomes cold from previously hot.

151. **A-T, B-T, C-T, D-T, E-T**
Usually aneurysmal bone cyst is primary tumour and arises secondary to venous obstruction or an AVF secondary to trauma. It can arise secondary to many other primary bone tumours due to hemodynamic changes. Other tumours associated are chondromyxoid fibroma, fibrous dysplasia, giant cell tumour, simple bone cyst, chondrosarcoma and osteosarcoma.

152. **A-T, B-T, C-T, D-T, E-T**
Tendon rupture may also be seen.

11 Haematological Lesions

1. Eosinophilia is seen in:
   A. Polyarteritis nodosa
   B. Hodgkin's disease
   C. Extrinsic allergic alveolitis
   D. Crohn's disease
   E. Hydatid bone

2. Hereditary spherocytosis:
   A. Autosomal recessive
   B. 1/100000 incidence
   C. Paraspinal masses seen in chest X-ray
   D. Presents above 40 years
   E. Ultrasound may show focal hyperechoic masses in the spleen

3. Histiocytosis:
   A. Skeletal survey should be done once clinical diagnosis is made
   B. Common in females
   C. 4-8 years is the peak incidence
   D. Hands and feet are rarely involved
   E. Birbeck granules should be seen to confirm pathological diagnosis

4. Well-defined lytic lesion with sclerotic margin, with no periosteal reaction is seen in:
   A. Histiocytosis   B. Metastases
   C. Hemangioma   D. Fibrous dysplasia
   E. Nonossifying fibroma

5. Histiocytosis:
   A. Punched out lesions are seen in the skull
   B. Bevelled edges are seen and pathognomonic
   C. Button sequestrum
   D. Floating teeth in lytic lesion is pathognomonic of mandibular histiocytosis
   E. Mastoid involvement is indistinguishable from mastoiditis

6. **Differential diagnosis of vertebra plana:**
   A. Gaucher's
   B. Lymphoma
   C. Histiocytosis
   D. Hemangioma
   E. Trauma

7. **Hodgkin's lymphoma:**
   A. Lymph node calcification is seen before treatment
   B. Septal lines are seen in chest X-ray
   C. CT shows mediastinal fibrosis after radiotherapy
   D. Regional lymph nodes are very commonly involved in primary bone lymphoma
   E. Most common location of bone lymphoma is the sternum secondary to mediastinal involvement

8. **Multiple myeloma:**
   A. Anaemia is normochromic normocytic
   B. Alkaline phosphatase is usually raised
   C. Bone scanning is very helpful
   D. Bone marrow aspirate may be normal
   E. Bence Jones protein is seen in urine in 80% of cases

9. **Multiple myeloma:**
   A. Increased incidence of bronchogenic carcinoma
   B. Carpal tunnel syndrome is a clinical feature
   C. Proximal myopathy is a recognized feature
   D. Hyperuricosuria occurs in the absence of treatment
   E. Normal bone scan virtually excludes the diagnosis

10. **Sickle cell anemia:**
    A. Hair on end skull is characteristic
    B. Hand and feet changes are not prominent
    C. Salmonella osteomyelitis is a recognized complication
    D. Avascular necrosis of the femoral head does not occur till the closure of the epiphysis
    E. In severe disease, splenomegaly is very common

11. **Mastocytosis:**
    A. 70% have bone involvement
    B. Diagnosed by finding mast cells in the tissues
    C. Mast cells are seen in the peripheral blood
    D. Urticaria pigmentosa is seen in 90%
    E. Increased renal size is commonly seen

12. **Features of mastocytosis:**
    A. Small bowel nodules   B. Lymphadenopathy
    C. Sclerotic bone lesions   D. Osteolytic lesions
    E. Trabecular thickening

13. **Myelosclerosis:**
    A. Causes leukoerythroblastic picture in peripheral smear
    B. Symmetrical periosteal reaction is seen in the femoral shaft
    C. Paraspinal soft tissue can be seen without spinal collapse
    D. Splenomegaly is seen occasionally
    E. Can be purely osteosclerotic

14. **Myelosclerosis is associated with:**
    A. Periosteal reaction along femur
    B. Increased density of the bone only
    C. Lytic lesions of the bone
    D. Sideroblastic anemia
    E. Lymphadenopathy

15. **Polycythemia rubra vera:**
    A. Splenomegaly is common
    B. Increased WBC count is seen
    C. Classically results in avascular necrosis
    D. Decreased oxygen-carrying capacity is seen
    E. Increased risk of peptic ulcer

16. **Eosinophilic granuloma:**
    A. Crosses the epiphysis
    B. Associated with periosteal reaction
    C. Fracture is presenting feature in 80%
    D. Associated with soft tissue mass
    E. Calcification

17. **Hurler's disease has the following features:**
    A. Stippled epiphyses
    B. Keratin sulphate in urine
    C. Heart failure
    D. Normal mental function
    E. Platyspondyly is the hall mark

18. **Mucopolysaccharidosis:**
    A. Hurler's is due to deficiency of iduronidase
    B. Hunter's is an autosomal recessive
    C. Keratan sulfate accumulates in Morquio's disease
    D. Morquio's is an autosomal dominant
    E. Mental retardation is severe in Hurler's

19. **Hurler's disease:**
    A. Mental retardation is a salient finding
    B. Facial features are coarse
    C. Tongue is atrophic
    D. Splenomegaly is seen
    E. Death is due to airway obstruction

20. **Features of Hurler's syndrome:**
    A. V shaped distal radius and ulna
    B. Bullet shaped fingers
    C. Hydrocephalus
    D. Superior beaking of vertebra
    E. Iliac flaring

21. **Features of Morquio's disease:**
    A. Mental retardation
    B. J-shaped sella
    C. Hook-shaped vertebra
    D. Metacarpals are wider than normal
    E. Flaring of iliac wings

22. **Features of Turner's syndrome:**
    A. Cubitus varus
    B. More common in metacarpals than phalanges
    C. Short 2nd and 5th middle phalanx
    D. Acro-osteolysis
    E. Calcification of epiphysis

23. **Causes of Madelung's deformity:**
    A. Ellis-van Creveld syndrome
    B. Spondyloepiphyseal dysplasia
    C. Turner's syndrome
    D. Diaphyseal aclasia
    E. Ollier's disease

24. **Madelung's deformity:**
    A. The essential deformity is growth retardation of medial portion of distal ulnar epiphysis
    B. The distal end of radius is inclined in palmar direction
    C. The lunate is tilted in the interosseous space
    D. The ulna is longer than radius
    E. The interosseous space is smaller than normal

25. **Madelung's deformity:**
    A. Reversed Madelung's deformity is seen in Ollier's disease
    B. Isolated Madelung's deformity is an X-linked disease

C. In reversed deformity, the distal end of radius is tiled dorsally and ulna displaced volarly

D. Wrist movements are not affected in Madelung's deformity

E. Usually bilaterally seen

F. More common in girls

26. **Cleidocranial dysostosis:**
    A. Specifically affects bones formed from membrane
    B. Acro-osteolysis is a recognised feature
    C. The femoral epiphysis shows lateral notching
    D. Cone-shaped epiphysis in middle phalanges
    E. Fusion of pubic symphysis

27. **Cleidocranial dysostosis:**
    A. Typically autosomal dominant
    B. Restricted mobility of shoulders
    C. Hearing is affected
    D. Wormian bones are seen
    E. The inner third of clavicle is absent

28. **Skeletal dysplasias:**
    A. In hypochondroplasia, trident hands are not seen like achondroplasia
    B. Interpediculate distance is normal in achondrogenesis
    C. Spinal canal narrowing is the hallmark of achondroplasia
    D. Homozygous achondroplasia die within a few days of life
    E. Homozygous achondroplasia resembles thanatophoric dysplasia

29. **Hypoplasia of maxillary antrum is seen in:**
    A. Kartagener's syndrome
    B. Paget's
    C. Thalassemia
    D. Down's
    E. Sickle cell disease

30. **Osteopetrosis:**
    A. The radiological findings in the congenital type and delayed type are essentially the same
    B. The cortex and medulla cannot be differentiated in long bones
    C. Bone within bone appearance is seen in 75% of cases
    D. Both transverse and longitudinal striations are seen
    E. Progressive improvement occurs in the type associated with renal tubular acidosis

31. **Hypoplasia of maxillary antrum is associated with:**
    A. Infraorbital margin is low
    B. Lateral wall of the nasal cavity is displaced laterally
    C. Thinning of antrum wall
    D. Enlarged orbit
    E. Low orbital floor

32. **Neurofibromatosis:**
    A. Dural ectasia is a recognized finding
    B. Pulsatile exophthalmos is caused due to sphenoid wing dysplasia
    C. Calcification can occur in the pareito-occipital area
    D. Posterior lumbar vertebral scalloping
    E. Increase in size during pregnancy

33. **Scoliosis:**
    A. Idiopathic scoliosis is the most common deformity seen in the spinal clinic
    B. Idiopathic scoliosis less than 70 degrees is not treated
    C. Sharp curve produces more deformity than smooth gentle curve
    D. Thoracic curves produce more deformity than lumbar curves
    E. Scoliosis is maximum in the morning than in the afternoon

34. **Scoliosis:**
    A. At least 10 degree of rotation should be present to qualify for scoliosis
    B. At least 5 degree of change in angle should be present to say that scoliosis has progressed
    C. Trunk rotation of more than 7 degree is abnormal
    D. MRI is routinely indicated for all patients with scoliosis
    E. Rotational deformities are best assessed by CT scan

35. **Features of neurofibromatosis:**
    A. Empty orbit
    B. Short curve scoliosis
    C. Growth disturbance leading to bone hypoplasia
    D. Beak deformity of L2
    E. Sesamoid index more than 40

36. **Neurofibromatosis:**
    A. Sporadic rather than hereditary
    B. Café au lait spots are present in less than 25%
    C. Associated with renal cell carcinoma
    D. Mixed enhancement pattern
    E. Anterior scalloping of vertebral bodies is common

37. **Pyknodysostosis:**
    A. Autosomal recessive inheritance
    B. The mandibular angle is obtuse
    C. The distal end of clavicle is not affected unlike osteopetrosis
    D. Acro-osteolysis is a characteristic feature
    E. Delayed closure of fontanelles is very common

38. **Osteopetrosis:**
    A. Not compatible with survival into old age
    B. Genetic in origin
    C. Increased risk of leukemia
    D. Normal healing of fractures
    E. Skull vault is usually involved

39. **Osteopetrosis:**
    A. Splenomegaly is associated
    B. Cranial nerve palsies are recognized complications
    C. Cannot be diagnosed in utero
    D. All the types of osteopetrosis are autosomal dominant
    E. There is an association with renal tubular acidosis

40. **Melorheostosis is associated with:**
    A. Neurofibromatosis   B. Tuberous sclerosis
    C. Osteopathia striata   D. Hemangioma
    E. Scleroderma

41. **Osteopathia striata:**
    A. Increased uptake is seen in bone scans
    B. Bilateral involvement
    C. The lines are transverse
    D. Epiphyseal involvement is very common
    E. The longest line is seen in tibia

42. **Dysplasias:**
    A. Osteopathia striata is autosomal dominant
    B. Melorheostosis is autosomal recessive
    C. Osteopathia striata is associated with osteopetrosis
    D. Multiple bone islands are seen in melorheostosis
    E. In melorheostosis there is normal uptake in scintigrams

43. **Melorheostosis:**
    A. Presents in infancy
    B. There are periods of exacerbation and remission
    C. Bilaterally symmetrical
    D. Upper limbs more common than lower limbs
    E. Starts proximally and extends distally

44. **Osteopetrosis:**
    A. Precocious type causes stillbirth
    B. Cartilaginous portion of skull base spared
    C. Hair on end skull is a feature
    D. Thickening of skull spares the inner table
    E. There is delayed myelination in brain

45. **Melorheostosis:**
    A. Flat bones are not affected
    B. Follows both sides of any long bone
    C. Causes premature epiphyseal closure
    D. There is no functional limitation of joint motion
    E. The medullary cavity is not encroached since it is a periosteal new bone

46. **Mafucci's syndrome:**
    A. Multiple osteochondromas
    B. Colonic polyps
    C. Multiple AVMs
    D. Hereditary predisposition
    E. 80% chances of malignant transformation

47. **Achondroplasia is associated with:**
    A. Champagne glass pelvis
    B. Posterior vertebral scalloping
    C. Spinal canal stenosis
    D. Small pituitary fossa
    E. Large foramen magnum

48. **Autosomal dominant inheritance is seen:**
    A. Achondroplasia
    B. Cystic fibrosis
    C. Adult polycystic renal disease
    D. Sickle cell disease
    E. Neurofibromatosis

49. **Spondyloepiphyseal dysplasia:**
    A. There is universal platyspondyly
    B. Cleft palate is associated
    C. Myopia is associated
    D. Disc height maintained like in Morquio's disease
    E. Epiphyses are irregular

50. **Ellis-van Creveld syndrome:**
    A. Hypoplastic nails and VSD are common
    B. Polydactyly is constantly seen in hands
    C. Drumstick appearance of proximal end of ulna

D. Hypoplastic lateral aspect of proximal tibia
E. Carpal fusion and premature ossification of proximal femoral epiphysis

51. **Asphyxiating thoracic dystrophy:**
    A. Rose thorn-shaped pelvis is characteristic
    B. Pulmonary hypoplasia is the most common cause of death in adults
    C. Renal failure is more common than in Ellis-van Creveld syndrome
    D. Associated with ASD
    E. Marked dysplasia in tibia

52. **Multiple epiphyseal dysplasia:**
    A. By definition, should include disturbance of more than one paired epiphyses
    B. The end plates are grossly irregular
    C. Tibiotalar slant is seen
    D. Manifests only when the child begins to walk
    E. With arms by side, fingertips reach midthigh

53. **Klippel-Feil syndrome is associated with:**
    A. Goldenhar's syndrome
    B. Cretinism
    C. Osteogenesis imperfecta
    D. Klippel-Trenaunay-Weber syndrome
    E. Assimilation of atlas

54. **Klippel-Feil syndrome:**
    A. Sprengel shoulder in 75%
    B. Deformed dens
    C. Spinal stenosis
    D. Duplication cysts
    E. VSD

55. **Klippel-Feil syndrome:**
    A. Only the anterior elements of the vertebra are fused
    B. The shape of the fused bone is altered
    C. The intervertebral disc space is not affected
    D. Intervertebral foramen is irregular
    E. Begins in C5-C7

56. **Common causes of acquired fusion of vertebra:**
    A. Trauma
    B. Tuberculosis
    C. Juvenile chronic arthritis
    D. Rheumatoid arthritis
    E. Reactive arthritis

57. **Radiological features of clubfoot:**
    A. The navicular bone is displaced laterally
    B. Metatarsals displaced medially
    C. Medial displacement of anterior calcaneum
    D. Hypertrophy of talar head
    E. Talar dome is flat

58. **Increase in size of lower limb is seen in:**
    A. Klippel-Trenaunay syndrome
    B. Lymphangioma
    C. Lipomatosis
    D. Neurofibromatosis
    E. Proteus syndrome

59. **Sprengel shoulder:**
    A. Always unilateral
    B. Omovertebral bone is often fibrous
    C. Increased incidence of clavicular fractures
    D. Omoclavicular bone is between clavicle and vertebra
    E. Omovertebral bone is usually from the superior border of the vertebral border of scapula

60. **Radiological features of Hurler's syndrome:**
    A. Changes in arms are more marked than changes in the legs
    B. Coxa vara
    C. Spina bifida
    D. J-shaped sella
    E. Platyspondyly

61. **Dysplasias:**
    A. In Polan's syndrome, serratus anterior is absent in chest wall
    B. Iliac horns are seen in nail patella syndrome
    C. In TAR syndrome, radius is fractured
    D. In Holt-Oram syndrome, thumb is absent and associated with ASD
    E. Holt-Oram syndrome is bilaterally symmetrical

62. **Melorheostosis:**
    A. Patellar dislocation is seen
    B. The radiological change is produced due to periosteal reaction
    C. Soft tissue is not affected
    D. Follows sclerotomal distribution
    E. MRI shows low signal in all sequences

63. **Osteogenesis imperfecta:**
    A. Can be diagnosed antenatally
    B. Usually fatal in utero
    C. Characteristically associated with deafness
    D. 60% incidence in the next born child
    E. Healing fractures show a florid callus formation

64. **Osteopoikilosis:**
    A. Skin changes are seen in form of keloid
    B. Common in the midshaft of any bone
    C. Presence of lucency within the lesion excludes the diagnosis
    D. The lesions are always less than 10 mm
    E. No uptake in bone scan
    F. Associated with Ollier's syndrome

65. **The following are skeletal dysplasias with decreased bone density:**
    A. Achondroplasia
    B. Osteogenesis imperfecta
    C. Homocystinuria
    D. Marfan's syndrome
    E. Menke's syndrome

66. **Dysplasias:**
    A. In Mafucci's syndrome, there is a correlation between the distribution of hemangiomas and enchondromas
    B. In metachondromatosis, there are multiple chondromas and exostoses
    C. In spondyloepiphyseal dysplasia tarda, the disc space is thin anteriorly and wide posteriorly
    D. Early and severe degeneration is seen in spondyloepiphyseal dysplasia
    E. Hyperostotic bone is deposited in the posterior two-thirds of end plate

67. **Trevor's disease (Dysplasia epiphysealis hemimelia):**
    A. Bilateral symmetrical
    B. Medial aspect of epiphysis affected more than lateral mass
    C. Metaphysis is unaffected
    D. The classical type is confined to single lower extremity
    E. After maturity, fuse with normal bone

68. **Diaphyseal aclasis:**
    A. Unlike solitary exostosis, in this exostosis points towards the joint
    B. Arises from epiphysis which is expanded
    C. Causes Madelung's deformity in wrist
    D. Fibula is shorter than normal
    E. Malignant transformation is seen in 3%

69. Scoliosis:
   A. Imaging is more extensively done in neurofibromatosis than muscular dystrophy
   B. Infantile scoliosis is scoliosis less than 1 year of age
   C. Infantile scoliosis requires surgery
   D. Infantile scoliosis is related to the way the child is positioned
   E. Infantile scoliosis is associated with skull and pelvic problems

70. Scoliosis:
   A. Cardiopulmonary complications are more common in early onset severe scoliosis
   B. Pulmonary complications are more in late onset scoliosis, if the curve is more than 100 degrees
   C. Up to 50% of scoliosis is idiopathic
   D. Apex vertebra is the one with the maximum rotation
   E. Stable vertebra is one which is nonrotated in the frontal film

71. Recognised causes of scoliosis:
   A. Osteoid osteoma
   B. Osteogenesis imperfecta
   C. Achondroplasia
   D. Duchenne's dystrophy
   E. Poliomyelitis

72. Scoliosis:
   A. Initial X-ray film should include the C7 and L1 vertebra
   B. Stagnaras view, is taken perpendicular to the true coronal plane of the apex vertebra
   C. Leeds lateral view is taken at 90 degrees to the Stagnaras view
   D. The iliac crest does not have to be necessarily included in the frontal film
   E. X-ray of the left hand is necessary

73. Differential diagnosis of osteolysis of bones:
   A. Leprosy
   B. Syringomyelia
   C. Scleroderma
   D. Pachydermoperiostitis
   E. Hypoparathyroidism

74. Features of Down's syndrome:
   A. Iliac index more than 60
   B. Acetabular angle less than 12 degrees
   C. Iliac angle less than 35 degrees
   D. Absent frontal sinus
   E. Incomplete ossification of manubrium sterni

75. **Features of Down's syndrome:**
    A. 13 pairs of ribs
    B. Lumbar vertebrae wider than taller
    C. Dolichocephaly
    D. The interorbital distance is shortened
    E. Contact sports to be avoided for fear of splenic rupture

76. **Skeletal dysplasias:**
    A. U-shaped vertebra is a feature of thanatophoric dwarfism
    B. Tibial excresecence is a feature of tuberous sclerosis
    C. Periosteal reaction in tuberous sclerosis is uncommon
    D. Telephone receiver appearance of tubular bones is a feature of achondrogenesis
    E. Thanatophoric dysplasia is associated with polyhydramnios

77. **Proximal femoral deficiency:**
    A. Unilateral in 90% of cases
    B. Increased incidence in diabetic mothers
    C. Aplasia of cruciate ligaments is associated
    D. It is not an inherited disease
    E. Acetabulum is deformed

78. **Enchondromatosis:**
    A. Multiple unilateral lesions are seen in Ollier's disease
    B. Multiple lipomas are seen in association with Mafucci's syndrome
    C. Calcification is characteristic
    D. Vertebral bodies are predominantly affected
    E. Lesions are mainly seen in flat bones

79. **Fibrous dysplasia:**
    A. Rib involvement can occur
    B. Accelerated epiphyseal fusion and sexual precocity occurs in males
    C. Infants have dense skull base
    D. Characteristic calcification is seen
    E. Polyostotic form is called Albers-Schönberg disease

80. **Achondroplasia:**
    A. Autosomal recessive inheritance
    B. Distal limb bones are commonly affected than proximal limb bones
    C. Sacrosciatic notches are wide
    D. Neurological symptoms may occur
    E. Lumbar spinal canal is stenosed

81. **Bone dysplasias with increased density:**
    A. Endosteal hyperostosis
    B. Diaphyseal dysplasia
    C. Caffey's disease
    D. Metaphyseal dysplasias
    E. Osteopoikilosis

82. **Achondroplasia:**
    A. The second common type of dwarfism
    B. There is gradual progression of deformities throughout life
    C. Mental development is never affected
    D. In hands there is widening of space between 3rd and 4th digits
    E. Causes transverse myelopathy

83. **Achondroplasia:**
    A. Death is due to narrow thorax
    B. Endochondral ossification is normal
    C. Progressive decrease of interpediculate distance in the lumbar vertebrae
    D. Disc space is typically narrowed
    E. Acetabula is vertically oriented

84. **Anomalies associated with maternal DM:**
    A. Craniolacunae
    B. Hirschsprung's
    C. Posterior urethral valve
    D. Anorectal atresia
    E. Patent ductus arteriosus

85. **Association of systemic (mastocytosis):**
    A. Hairy cell leukemia
    B. Polycythemia
    C. Castleman disease
    D. Non-Hodgkin's lymphoma
    E. Anemia

86. **Hemophilias:**
    A. 80% of haemophilias have their first bleed between 5-10 years
    B. Changes mimic those of Still's disease
    C. Autosomal recessive condition
    D. Pannus and erosions are seen
    E. Trabeculae-thinned

ANSWERS

1. **A-T, B-T, C-F, D-F, E-T**
   Seen in fungal and parasitic infections, connective tissue disease, tumours and allergies.

2. **A-F, B-F, C-T, D-F, E-T**
   1/5000 incidence. Focal hypoechoic infarcts are seen in the spleen. Hereditary spherocytosis is autosomal dominant. Paraspinal masses may be seen due to extramedullary haematopoiesis.

3. **A-T, B-F, C-F, D-T, E-T**
   Histiocytosis is common in males, 1-4 years; common in < 15 years. Skull, mandible, ribs, long bones, tibia, femur and humerus are commonly involved.
   Presence of Birbeck granules is essential for pathological diagnosis.

4. **A-T, B-T, C-T, D-T, E-T**
   Simple bone cyst, aneurysmal bone cyst, enchondroma, non-ossifying fibroma, fibrous dysplasia, healing metastases and intraosseous hemangioma are the common causes.

5. **A-T, B-T, C-T, D-T, E-T**
   Geographical appearance is seen in skull due to destruction of both tables by varying degrees. Jaw lesions are seen in 40% of multifocal histiocytosis. Alveolar margins affected.

6. **A-T, B-T, C-T, D-T, E-T**
   Metastasis is also a recognised cause. Eosinophilic granuloma is the most common cause in children.

7. **A-F, B-T, C-T, D-F, E-F**
   Hodgkin's nodes are usually hypodense and show moderate enhancement. Calcification is seen after radiotherapy or chemotherapy. Septal lines can be seen if there is pulmonary involvement. In primary bone lymphoma, bone is the only organ usually involved. The most common location of bone lymphoma is the spine.

8. **A-T, B-F, C-F, D-T, E-T**
   Bone scanning is not hot and is not usually helpful.

9. **A-F, B-T, C-T, D-T, E-F**
   MM is a rare cause of carpal tunnel syndrome.

10. **A-F, B-F, C-T, D-F, E-F**
    In severe disease, the spleen is atrophied due to multiple splenic infarcts. Avascular necrosis seen in femur, humerus, later than Perthes disease. Hair on end is seen, not as frequently as thalassemia. Salmonella is spread by bacteremia from bowel.

11. **A-T, B-T, C-F, D-T, E-F**

12. **A-T, B-T, C-T, D-T, E-T**
Mastocytosis systemic infiltration by mastocytes: Bones involved in 70%, skin is the most common organ. Diffuse osteosclerosis seen due to trabecular thickening. Ro nodular/round focal sclerosis may be seen. Focal osteolysis/sclerosis also seen. Hepatomegaly, splenomegaly, lymphadenopathy seen. Esophagitis/strictures, peptic ulcer, nodules/thick irregular folds in small intestine, polyps, diverticulosis, portal hypertension, Budd-Chiari sclerosing cholangitis, more common in children. In child, bones are not commonly affected.

13. **A-T, B-F, C-T, D-F, E-T**
Leukoerythroblastic picture is characteristic of myelosclerosis. Paraspinal soft tissue due to extramedullary hematopoiesis. Periosteal reaction not symmetrical. Splenomegaly 90%.

14. **A-T, B-F, C-T, D-F, E-T**
There is increased density in the spleen also. Normocytic normochromic anaemia is seen instead of the sideroblastic anemia.

15. **A-T, B-T, C-F, D-F, E-T**
Increased production of all cells. Splenomegaly 75%. Avascular necrosis can be seen due to capillary blockage by high viscous blood. CVA, myocardial infarction, peptic ulcer, mesenteric thrombosil, GI bleed, gout, myelofibrosis, leukemia, peripheral vascular disease are other complications.

16. **A-T, B-T, C-F, D-T, E-F**
Usually diaphyseal, lytic, may be expansile, ill-defined/sclerotic margins, cortical thinning, erosion of cortex, linear periosteal reaction, soft tissue, occasional pathological fractures. Mimic infection/tumour. Occasionally cross into epiphysis.

17. **A-F, B-F, C-T, D-F, E-F,**
Stippled epiphysis is a feature of chondrodysplasia punctata.
In Hurler's, there is increased excretion of dermatan sulfate and heparan sulfate in urine. Mental retardation is severe. Platyspondyly—features of Morquio's cardiomyopathy, cardiac failure seen.

18. **A-T, B-F, C-T, D-F, E-T**

IH—Hurler's AR	α L Iduronidase	Dermatan sulfate, heparan sulfate
IS—Schies	α L Iduronidase	Dermatan sulfate, heparan sulfate
IHS	α L Iduronidase	Dermatan sulfate, heparan sulfate
II Hunter's XR	Iduronate sulfatase	Dermatan sulfate, heparan sulfate

III San Filippo	A heparan sulfatase	
	B α N acetyl glucosaminidase	heparan sulfate
	C Acetyl CoA α glucosaminidase N acetyl transferase	
	D n acetyl glucosamine 6 sulfate sulfatase	
IV Morquio—AR	A Galactosamine 6 sulfate sulfatase	Keratan sulfate
	B α Galactosamine	
VI marateaux	Aryl sulfatase	Dermatan sulfate
Lamy		
VII Sly	α Glucuronidase	Dermatan sulfate
VIII Diferrante	Glucosamine 6 sulfate sulfatase	Dermatan sulfate

19. **A-T, B-T, C-F, D-T, E-T**

Mental retardation is seen, but not at birth. Gargolysism is seen. Splenomegaly, hepatomegaly, cardiomegaly, umbilical hernia and hypertension are seen. Tongue is large. Death is due to congestive cardiac failure or airway obstruction which can be due to infiltration of larynx, trachea, adenoids, high epiglottis, abnormal cervical spine, abnormal chest motion.

20. **A-T, B-T, C-T, D-F, E-T**

The radiological findings of Hurler's are those of dysostosis multiplex which are seen in most of mucopolysaccharidosis and mucolipidosis. Skull—large, dolichocephaly, thick diploic space, J-shaped sella, hypoplastic mastoids and sinuses, flat condyle, malformed teeth, large tongue and adenoids, Spine—kyphoscoliosis, beaking, (middle—Morquio's, inferior—Hurler's) flat vertebra. Pelvis—wide acetabular roof, wide acetabular angle, iliac flaring, wide femoral neck, dysplastic femoral neck. Chest—short wide clavicles, wide ribs. Long bones—delayed ossification, varus, Hand—V-shaped distal radius, ulna, small carpals, Bullet fingers—proximal tapering of metacarpals and phalanges. Brain—hydrocephalus, loss of grey white matter differentiation, delayed myelination. Mental retardation mild in Hunters, normal intelligence in Morquio's.

21. **A-F, B-T, C-T, D-F, E-T**

Morquio-Brailsford disease is a mucopolysaccharidosis, without mental retardation. The affected person is short. Skull is large, elongated, with J-shaped sella. Characteristic finding is platyspondyly, with middle beaking. Metacarpals are short and have proximal tapering. Phalanges also taper peripherally. Coxa valga, narrow femoral neck, hypoplasia acetabulum, hypoplastic capital femoral epiphysis and odontoid hypoplasia are other features.

22. **A-F, B-F, C-T, D-F, E-F**

Cubitus valgus, common in phalanges than metacarpals, positive metacarpal and carpal sign. Swollen drumstick distal phalanges, epiphysis insetting into the bases of adjacent metaphysis.

23. **A-F, B-F, C-T, D-T, E-T**
Multiple epiphyseal dysplasia, dyschondrosteosis, trauma and infection are other causes.

24. **A-F, B-T, C-T, D-T, E-F**
Madelung's deformity is caused due to retardation of growth of the medial portion of the distal radial epiphysis. The radius is bowed laterally and dorsally, with ulnar and palmar inclination of the distal end. The distal end of ulna is undeveloped, longer than radius and ulnar head is enlarged and dorsally placed. The interosseous space is wide. The distal end of radius and ulna form a V shape and the carpal bones occupy this space. The ulnate is at the apex, scaphoid radially and triquetrum on the ulnar side. The carpals are shifted to the ulnar and volar side.

25. **A-T, B-F, C-T, D-F, E-T, F-T**
In reversed Madelung's deformity, the plane of the distal end of articular surface is reversed, and hence the carpus is shifted towards the dorsal side. Isolated Madelung's deformity is autosomal dominant, bilateral and common in males. Wrist movement is affected, supination more than pronation.

26. **A-T, B-T, C-T, D-T, E-F**
Specifically affects ossification of membranous bones and associated with midline defects. The pubic symphysis is widely separated.

27. **A-T, B-F, C-T, D-T, E-F**
Cleidocranial dysostosis is typically autosomal dominant, but can be autosomal recessive. The clavicle is hypoplastic or absent or pseudoarthrosis and is common in the lateral third of clavicle. There is increased mobility of the shoulder joint. Hearing is affected due to sclerosis of the mastoid and petrous portions of the temporal bone. Wormian bone, peristent metopic suture, delayed ossification of calvarium and delayed closure of fontanelles are features.

28. **A-T, B-T, C-T, D-T, E-T**
Hypochondroplasia is a less severe, autosomal dominant disease. Achondrogenesis is an autosomal recessive disease with defective ossification, especiallly of vertebral bodies and skull with metaphyseal spur.

29. **A-T, B-T, C-T, D-T, E-F**
Thalassemia, Cretinism, Kartagener's syndrome, Down's syndrome, Paget's disease and fibrous dysplasis are the common causes of hypoplasia of maxillary antrum.

30. **A-T, B-T, C-F, D-T, E-T**
    Radiological findings in congenital and delayed type are similar, except that the delayed type shows milder changes. The bones are sclerotic, the cortex and medulla cannot be differentiated. Bone within bone appearance is characteristic but is unusual. The miniature central bones are primitive, fibrillar and cellular osseous tissue separated from cortex by nonsclerotic bone or rudimentally medullary cavity. Metaphysis is club shaped. Mottled lucent areas can be seen. Longitudinal striations are uncommon and are sites of blood vessels. Transverse striations are alternating areas of mature bone and intensely sclerotic disorganised osseous tissue.

31. **A-T, B-T, C-F, D-T, E-T**
    Antral wall is thickened.

32. **A-T, B-T, C-T, D-T, E-T**
    Splenoid using dysplasia seen in 5-10%. Hamartomas, tumour are seen in CNS. Other findings are kyphoscoliosis, spondylolisthesis, meningoceles, neurofibromas, enlarged spinal foramina, pseudo-arthrosis, macrocephaly thinned cortex. Increased size and number during pregnancy.

33. **A-T, B-F, C-T, D-T, E-F**
    Idiopathic scoliosis less than 40 degree is usually not corrected. A five degree diurnal variation can be normally seen and is maximum in the afternoon.

34. **A-F, B-F, C-T, D-F, E-T**
    Five degree rotation is enough to confirm scoliosis, but 10 degree change is required to confirm progression. Trunk rotation is measured by scoliometer and a 7 degree rotation, corresponding to 20 degrees in Cobb's measurement is significant. The role of MRI is controversial in scoliosis. But it should be done in all atypical cases, to exclude other causes of scoliosis, to find associated anomalies. It is especially done before surgery. If MRI is not done before surgery, assessment of spine by MRI after surgery might be rendered difficult due to the surgical device.

35. **A-T, B-T, C-T, D-F, E-F**
    Bare orbit due to sphenoid using dysplasia. Sharp curve scoliosis is a feature of neurofibromatosis. Sesamoid index = product of diameter of medial sesamoid in I MCP joints in two views, > 32 in women and > 40 in men indicate acromegaly.

36. **A-T, B-F, C-F, D-F, E-F**
    Café au lait spots seen in 95%.
    Posterior scalloping of vertebra is seen, but there is no anterior scalloping. Association with renal artery stenosis/aneurysms and pheochromocytoma.

37. **A-T, B-T, C-F, D-T, E-T**

Pyknodysostosis is autosomal recessive unlike many other structural anomalies. Wide sutures, wormian bones, small maxilla, poorly developed mastoids, malformed teeth, dense orbits, sclerotic skull base and thin vault, increased density of vertebra, resorption of distal end of clavicles and terminal phalanges, short hands and osteosclerosis of long bones are characteristic features. Pathological fractures, osteomyelitis and sleep apnoea are common complications.

38. **A-T, B-T, C-T, D-T, E-T**

39. **A-T, B-T, C-F, D-F, E-F**

There are many types of osteopetrosis. The precocious type is autosomal recessive and is lethal. The delayed type, also called Albers-Schönberg' disease is autosomal dominant. Intermediate type is autosomal recessive. The association with renal tubular acidosis is called Sly's disease or marble brain disease. Cranial nerve palsies are very common complications, with optic nerve and acoustic nerve affected commonly producing deafness and blindness.

40. **A-T, B-T, C-T, D-T, E-T**

Also associated with osteopoikilosis and AVM.

41. **A-F, B-T, C-F, D-T, E-T**

Osteopathia striata is characterised by presence of vertical lines, usually in metaphysis extending to the diaphysis and very rarely into the epiphysis. This is believed to be due to bone remodelling. The length of the line depends on the rate of the growth of the bone. There is no increased uptake in bone scans. In pelvis there is a fan-like pattern, called sunburst effect extending from acetabulum to the iliac crest.

42. **A-T, B-F, C-T, D-T, E-F**

Melorheostosis is not inherited and the etiology is unknown yet. The bone scan shows increased uptake in the abnormal areas unlike osteopathia striata which show normal uptake.

43. **A-F, B-T, C-F, D-F, E-T**

Melorheostosis presents in late childhood or adolescence. It is monomelic, affecting lower limb more common than upper limb. It has a slow course.

44. **A-T, B-F, C-T, D-F, E-T**

The precocious type is the lethal congenital type, inherited in AR fashion. It can cause stillbirth. The skull is thickened with both inner and outer tables affected, with hair on end apearance, with involvement of cartilaginous portion. Mastoids and sinuses are poorly developed. Teeth are malformed and cranial nerve foramen are narrow. Brain shows delayed myelination, optic nerve atrophy, hydrocephalus and calcification in basal ganglia.

45. **A-F, B-F, C-T, D-F, E-F**
Melorheostosis has a typical waxy flowing cortical thickening, along one side of a long bone. In adults it is mainly periosteal and does not involve the medullary cavity, but in children it is mainly endosteal and narrows the medullary cavity. It can affect scapula, vertebra, ribs, skull and facial bones. It can cause limitation of joint motion, genu varum, valgus foot and patellar dislocation. Deformities can be seen.

46. **A-F, B-F, C-F, D-F, E-F**
Mafucci's syndrome combination of multiple enchondromas and hemangiomas. Most are sporadic, men>women. Asymmetrical 40-50% chance of chondrosarcoma. Angiosarcoma can arise.

47. **A-T, B-T, C-T, D-T, E-F**
The foramen magnum is constricted in achondroplasia.

48. **A-T, B-F, C-T, D-F, E-T**

49. **A-T, B-T, C-T, D-F, E-T**
There are two types AD and AR. AD manifests at birth, but AR presents later. There is also a lethal subtype. The vertebrae show kyphoscoliosis. The vertebrae are flattened, but the disc height appears increased, unlike Morquio's where it is maintained and there is central beaking. The vertebrae are pear shaped in infancy due to lack of development of posteior portion or trapexoid shaped. Odontoid hypoplasia, short scapulae, absent stenral ossification centers, short iliac wings, horizontal acetabular roof and delayed epiphyseal ossification are other features.

50. **A-T, B-T, C-T, D-T, E-T**
Also called chondroectodermal dysplasia. Characterised by absent or hypoplastic nails, dwarfism, polydactyly, cardiac anomalies (VSD, single atrium). Tibial plateau changes are characteristic with widened metaphysis, eostosis from medial end. There is also drumstick appearance of distal end of radius. Polydactyly is uncommon in feet.

51. **A-T, B-F, C-T, D-F, E-F**
Also called Jeune's syndrome, characterised by short horizontal ribs with high handle bar clavicle producing small thoracic cavity. Pulmonary hypoplasia is the cause of death in children and renal

failure in adults. Polydactyly is less common and inconstant. Cardiac changes and nail changes are not seen. Epiphyseal changes are not seen. Pelvis has the rose thorn or triradiate appearance, with a flat downward spike at medial, lateral and cenetral aspect of acetabular roof. This can normalise with age.

52. **A-F, B-F, C-T, D-T, E-T**

By definition, more than two paired epiphysis are affected, with irregular epiphyseal growth, especially in hips, knees and ankles. There is only minimal irregularity of endplates. The disease manifests when child begins to walk. There is short stature due to lower limb involvement. In a normal person, the fingertips reach the level of greater trochanter. But here, they reach midthigh. Many deformities are associated including coxa vara, genu valgum and varum. Tibiotalar slant is deformity of lateral portion of distal tibial epiphysis and is also seen in JRA and hemophilia.

53. **A-T, B-T, C-T, D-F, E-T**

54. **A-F, B-T, C-T, D-T, E-T**

There are many associated features of Klippel-Feil syndrome. Others include cervical ribs, spina bifida, hemivertebra, webbed neck, kyphoscoliosis, deformed ribs, cranial asymmetry, cleft palate, supernumery lung lobes, patent foramen ovale, enteric cysts. Sprengel's shoulder is seen only in 25%. The characteristic clinical triad of Klippel-Feil syndrome is short neck, low posterior hair line and limitation of movements of neck.

55. **A-F, B-T, C-F, D-T, E-F**

Klippel-Feil syndrome produces vertebral fusion which should be differentiated from acquired fusion. This affects both anterior and posterior elements. Trapezoidal shape of fused segment due to chronicity and remodelling, small calcified intervertebral disc, and irregular intervertebral foramina. In acquired fusion, only the anterior element is affected, no change in shape of vertebra, normal disc height and IV foramen. It usually begins in occiput-C1 or C1-2 or C2.

56. **A-T, B-T, C-T, D-F, E-F**

Ankylosing spondylitis and surgery are other recognised causes.

57. **A-F, B-T, C-T, D-T, E-T**

Navicular bone is oriented medially and inferiorly. Internal tibial torsion is another feature.

58. **A-T, B-T, C-F, D-T, E-T**

KT syndrome part wire stain, soft tissue, bone hypertrophy, venous malformation proteus syndrome—Hamartoma, partial gigantism, vascular malformation, lipoma, nevi macrodystrophia lipomatosa affects only foot. DVT, trauma, compartment syndrome, infections are acquired causes.

59. **A-F, B-T, C-F, D-F, E-F**
Sprengel's shoulder is elevation of scapula, which can be unilateral or bilateral. It is seen in 25% of Klippel-Feil syndrome. Omovertebral bone is from the middle of inferior portion of the vertebral border of scapula to the vertebra and this can be osseous cartilaginous, fibrous or a true joint. Omoclavicular bone is between the scapula and clavicle.

60. **A-T, B-F, C-F, D-T, E-F**
Features of dysostosis multiplex.

61. **A-F, B-T, C-F, D-T, E-T**
Poland's syndrome—absence of sternal portion of pectoralis major and pectoralis minor.
TAR syndrome—thrombocytopenia, absent radius. Hand deviated medially.
Holt-Oram syndrome—bilaterally symmetrical, absent thumb or three phalanges in thumb, with ASD/VSD/anomalous great vessels.

62. **A-T, B-F, B-F, D-T, E-T**
The waxy bone is mature haversian bone with osteoids and fibrous tissue. Waxy appearance due to endosteal bone proliferation. Usually lower limb, can reach foot associated with NF, scleroderma, osteopoikilosis, osteopathia striata, tuberous sclerosis.

63. **A-T, B-F, C-T, D-F, E-T**
OI—There are four types, I—Mild, survive till old age, dentition normal IA; abnormal IB, hearing impairment II—lethal stillborn, blue sclera is seen, III rare severe die by 30 years, abnormal teeth, blue sclera IV—mild-moderately severe, survive till old age, no blue sclera, IVA normal dentition, B abnormal kyphoscoliosis, pseudoarthrosis, wormian bones, basilar invagination, metaphyseal lesions, osteoporosis and cod fish vertebra.

64. **A-T, B-F, C-F, D-T, E-T**
This is an autosomal dominant disease. It is usually seen after three years in males. Cutaneous changes include keloid and scleroderma like lesions. There are multiple, 1-10 mm foci of bone, which are made of compact lamellar bone with haversian system. They are typically seen in the juxta-articular region in the epiphyseal and metaphyseal region. In the pelvis they are seen in the acetabulum and in the shoulder they are close to the glenoid. Longitudinal

striations can be seen. Associated with osteopathia striata and osteosarcoma. Associated with Buschke-Ollendorff syndrome (High elastik in dermis).

65. A-F, B-T, C-T, D-F, E-T
Idiopathic juvenile osteoporosis is another recognised cause.

66. A-F, B-T, C-T, D-T, E-T
In metachondromatosis, osteochondroma points towards joints.

67. A-F, B-T, C-F, D-T, E-T
This is a unilateral, irregular enlargement of the medial or lateral portion of one or more epiphysis on one side of the body. The classicial type is confined to a single lower extremity. Monostotic form is localised. Generalised form affects entire lower extremity. The bony mass covered with epiphyseal cartilage is attached to the remainder of epiphysis, sometimes separate from the epiphysis. They can either fuse with normal bone at maturity or persist as separate bodies. Metaphyseal changes can be seen secondary to epiphyseal changes.

68. A-F, B-F, C-T, D-T, E-T
Diaphyseal aclasis is multiple cartilage capped exostosis near the diaphyseal side of physeal line in the metaphysis. The exostosis points away from the epiphysis. The metaphysis is expanded. This continues to grow till epiphyseal fusion. Bone destruction at the base of exostosis, irregularity and changing appearance of calcification indicate malignant conversion.

69. A-T, B-F, C-F, D-T, E-T
Imaging is more extensive in conditions such as neurofibromatosis and congenital deformities. Infantile scoliosis is less than 3 years, juvenile 4-10 years and adolescent after 10 years. Infantile scoliosis is associated with developmental problems and may be related to the position of the child in the cot. It resolves spontaneously and does not require surgery.

70. A-T, B-F, C-T, D-T, E-F
Early onset scoliosis (< 5 years), if severe, results in more cardiopulmonary complications rather than the late onset scoliosis, where the complications are less even if the curve is more than 100 degrees. Up to 80% is idiopathic and 10% are congenital. The apex vertebra is the one with the maximum rotation. The stable vertebra is the one which is bisected by the midsacral line. Neutral vertebra is nonrotated in plain film.

71. A-T, B-T, C-F, D-T, E-T
Causes of scoliosis are idiopathic, congenital defects in bone formation (wedge, blocked, hemi and fused verebra) and neuro-

logical defects (tethered cord, meningocele, diastomatomyelia, synringomyelia, Chiari), neuromuscular (cerebral palsy, spinocerebellar degeneration, polio, Duchenne's, congenital hypotonia), developmental (OI, NF, dysplasias) and tumour related (osteoid osteoma, osteoblastoma, spinal cord tumours).

72. **A-F, B-T, C-T, D-F, E-T**
Frontal and lateral films from the lower cervical level up to the sacral level, including the iliac crests are obligatory. The other derotated views may be done. Iliac crest should be included for the Risser's index. X-ray left hand is required to find out the bone age and indicates severe future deformity if the bone age is less than expected.

73. **A-T, B-T, C-T, D-T, E-F**
Hyperparathyroidism, pyknodysostosis, progeria, epidermolysis bullosa, syringomyelia, syphilis, leprosy, psoriasis and vinyl chloride are other causes of osteolysis. There are congenital forms including idiopathic osteolysis and Hadjdu-Cheney type of osteolysis.

74. **A-F, B-T, C-T, D-T, E-F**
Normal iliac index is more than 68, 60-68 is considered probable Down's and less than 60 is definite Down's syndrome. Iliac angle less than 35 degrees before 3 months and less than 45 degrees after 3 months is suggestive. There is extra ossification center for manubrium sterni. Other features include hyoplastic middle and distal phalanges, clinidactyly, short metacarpals, duodenal stenosis, Hirschsprung's disease.

75. **A-F, B-F, C-F, D-F, E-F**
There are 11 pairs of ribs. Lumbar vertebrae are taller than wider producing a cuboid shape. Brachycephaly is seen. The interorbital distance is increased and there is brachycephaly producing the Mongoloid face. Contact sports is avoided for fear of atlantoaxial instability.

76. **A-T, B-T, C-F, D-F, E-T**
Telephone receiver type of long bones is also a feature of thanatophoric dwarfism.
Tuberous sclerosis has a triad of mental retardation, seizures and skin lesions. Intracranial calcification, cysts and periosteal reaction in phalanges and discrete bone islands are other features.

77. **A-T, B-T, C-T, D-T, E-T**
The proximally deficient femur is displaced laterally, superiorly and posteriorly towards the iliac crest. The distal femur is usually

normal. Ossification of femoral head is delayed or absent. Varus deformity, femoral shaft shortening and agenesis of femoral head are noted. Secondary changes in acetabulum and pelvis will also be seen.

78. **A-T, B-F, C-T, D-F, E-F**
Enchondromas are seen in metaphysis of long bones and diaphysis of short tubular bones Ollier's is more common in long bones. 50% chance of malignant conversion. Calcification is progressive. Loss of calcification in focal region indicates malignant degeneration.

79. **A-T, B-F, C-T, D-F, E-F**
Accelerated epiphyseal fusion and precocity is common in females and is called McCune-Albright syndrome. Albers-Schönberg' is a type of osteopetrosis seen in adults.

80. **A-F, B-F, C-F, D-T, E-T**
Autosomal dominant inheritance. The proximal bones are shortened. Sacrosciatic notches are small. Neurological complications are very common due to spinal canal narrowing.

81. **A-T, B-T, C-T, D-F, E-T**
There are many dysplasias with increased bone density. Osteopetrosis, pyknodysostosis, dysosteosclerosis, osteosclerosis, osteopoikilosis, melorheostosis, osteopathia striata, craniodiaphyseal dysplasia, craniometaphyseal dysplasia, pachydermoperiostitis, frontometaphyseal dysplasia, Pyle's dysplasia, Caffey's disease.

82. **A-F, B-F, C-F, D-T, E-T**
It is the most common cause of dwarfism. The clinical and radiological manifestations are present at birth and do not change significantly during entire lifetime. Mental development is normally not affected, but if there is hydrocephalus, mental retardation can be seen. Can cause nerve root compression, spinal stenosis, acute transverse myelopathy.

83. **A-T, B-F, C-F, D-F, E-F**
Death can be due to brainstem compression by narrow foramen magnum or chest compression by narrow thorax. Endochondral ossification is typically affected. In normal persons, there is progressive increase of interpediculate distance from proximal to distal lumbar vertebrae. In achondroplasia, there is no increase, but there is no decrease. Disc space is increased due to excess cartilage. Acetabula is horizontally oriented.

84. **A-T, B-F, C-T, D-T, E-T**
    Cardiomyopathy, truncus arteriosus, double outlet right ventricle, renal agenesis, caudal regresion agenesis, DiGeorge anomaly CNS and pancreatic anomalies.

85. **A-T, B-T, C-T, D-T, E-T**
    Also associated with thrombocythemia, hypereosinophilic syndrome, monoclonal gammopathy. Anemia, eosinophilia, leukocytosis, basophilia, thrombocytosis, monocytosis are seen.

86. **A-F, B-T, C-F, D-T, E-F**
    70% have first bleed before 2 years. TB, JRA are common mimics X-linked recessive disease, seen only in males. Trabeculae are coarsened although they may be lost during osteopenia. Growth arrest lines, soft tissue density, hypertrophic synovium are other features.

Interventional Radiology

1. **Indications of vertebroplasty:**
   A. Radicular pain
   B. Fracture with retropulsed fragment
   C. Pain localised to fracture
   D. Cord compression
   E. Tuberculosis

2. **Vertebroplasty:**
   A. Posterolateral approach used for cervical vertebra
   B. Transpedicular approach used for thoracic vertebrae
   C. Procedure is successful only if entire vertebra is opacified
   D. Procedure aborted if paraspinous veins opacified
   E. The cement is mixed with tantalum

3. **Spinal biopsy:**
   A. Risk of fracture is increased after bone biopsy
   B. Anaesthesia can cause paralysis of motor nerve
   C. Motor nerve injury recovers in 3-4 hours
   D. Spinal cord compression does not occur in spinal biopsy
   E. Increased risk of spinal cord compression in biopsy of hypervascular tumours

4. **The following are contraindications for bone biopsy:**
   A. C1 lesion
   B. Lesion surrounded by infected tissue
   C. Odontoid process lesion
   D. Hemorrhagic lesions
   E. Pathological fracture

5. **Bone biopsy:**
   A. CT is preferred over fluoroscopy for deeper lesions
   B. Sclerotic lesions require Chiba needle or other small bore needles
   C. Destructive lesions usually require trephine needles
   D. Combination of aspiration and biopsy is synergistic
   E. Tru cut needles are of no use in bone biopsy

6. **Bone biopsy:**
   A. Transpedicular approach is not used if the medial pedicle wall is lost
   B. CSF leak is the major complication of transpedicular approach
   C. Biopsy through a fracture can be confused with malignancy
   D. The biopsy can be repeated up to three times only
   E. Yield is lower in sclerotic lesion than lytic lesion

7. **Vertebroplasty:**
   A. Antibiotic is given along with cement, if patient is immuno-suppressed
   B. Pulmonary embolism is a complication
   C. Spinal stenosis can result
   D. Pain relief is seen in 90%
   E. No more treatment for osteoporosis is required

8. **Bone biopsy:**
   A. Nickel needles are used for MRI-guided biopsy
   B. Carbon fiber needles are used for improved visualisation of needle in MRI-guided biopsy
   C. Frequency encoding direction is placed perpendicular to the plane of needle
   D. Higher incidence of complications in MRI-guided biopsy
   E. Biopsy should be avoided through myxoid areas in sarcoma

9. **The following are recognised associations:**
   A. Straight back syndrome and aortic stenosis
   B. Intramural diverticulosis and diabetes
   C. Posterior fossa tumour and pheochromocytoma
   D. Cholangiocarcinoma and contraceptive pills
   E. Café au lait spots and small orbits

10. **Recognised associations:**
    A. Medullary carcinoma of thyroid and neurofibromatosis
    B. Paroxysmal nocturnal hemoglobinuria and Budd-Chiari syndrome
    C. Esophageal atresia and Down's syndrome
    D. High-arched palate and arachnodactyly
    E. Amiodarone and cardiomyopathy

11. **The following are recognised associations:**
    A. Short 4th metacarpal and depressed medial tibial condyle
    B. Peutz-Jeghers syndrome and carcinoma of pancreas
    C. Acanthosis nigricans and carcinoma of pancreas
    D. Pemphigus vulgaris and esophageal strictures
    E. Enchondromas and sarcomas

12. **Complications of steroid therapy:**
    A. Acute pancreatitis
    B. Nephrocalcinosis
    C. Osteomalacia
    D. Skeletal muscle atrophy
    E. Mediastinal lipomatosis

13. **There is increased incidence of:**
    A. Bronchogenic carcinoma in a TB patient
    B. Stomach carcinoma in pernicious anaemia
    C. Bladder carcinoma in a smoker
    D. Pancreatic carcinoma in a diabetic
    E. Colonic carcinoma in juvenile polyps

14. **Associations:**
    A. Scleroderma and lung cancer
    B. Hemochromatosis and chondrocalcinosis
    C. Pseudomembranous colitis and ankylosing spondylitis
    D. Erosive arthropathy and primary biliary cirrhosis
    E. Cystic fibrosis and cirrhosis

15. **Phleboliths are seen in the following syndromes:**
    A. Mafucci's syndrome
    B. Marfan's syndrome
    C. Chondrocalcinosis
    D. Diverticulosis
    E. Orbital varix

16. **Malignancy is associated with:**
    A. Dermatitis herpetiformis
    B. Psoriasis
    C. Pemphigus
    D. Crohn's disease
    E. Epidermolysis bullosa

17. **Calcification in plain film:**
    A. Mottled renal calcification is likely to be RCC
    B. Hydatid in lung never calcifies
    C. Hepatoblastoma commonly calcifies
    D. Carcinoid of appendix calcifies frequently
    E. Calcification is seen in Klippel-Trenaunay syndrome

18. **Recognised associations:**
    A. Esophageal atresia and Down's syndrome
    B. Dissecting aneurysm and Marfan's syndrome
    C. Subarachnoid haemorrhage and coarctation of aorta
    D. Analgesic nephropathy and transitional cell carcinoma
    E. Superficial thrombophlebitis and Behçet's disease

19. **Increased incidence of carcinoma is seen in:**
    A. Peutz-Jeghers syndrome
    B. Cholecochal cyst
    C. Sclerosing cholangitis
    D. Celiac disease
    E. Ectopia vesicae

20. **Amyloidosis causes:**
    A. Small kidneys   B. Carpal tunnel syndrome
    C. Lobar pneumonia   D. Splenomegaly
    E. Alzheimer's dementia

21. **Features of phenytoin treatment:**
    A. Enlarged hilar lymphadenopathy
    B. Calvarial sclerosis
    C. Folate deficiency anaemia
    D. Thickened heel pad
    E. Nystagmus

22. **Radiological signs and their causes:**
    A. Celery stalk—Rubella infection
    B. Apple core—Polypoid colonic cancer
    C. Lemon sign—Arnold Chiari
    D. Banana sign—Spina bifida
    E. Hamburger sign—Facetal joint dislocation

23. **Radiological signs and their causes:**
    A. Linguine sign—extracapsular implant rupture
    B. Cottage loaf sign—diaphragmatic rupture
    C. Doughnut sign—testicular torsion
    D. Pancake vertebra—eosinophilic granuloma
    E. Draping aorta sign—acute rupture

24. **Radiological signs and their causes:**
    A. Pop corn calcification—fibroadenoma
    B. Licked candy stick appearance—leprosy
    C. Salt and pepper skull—hyperparathyroidism
    D. Champagne glass pelvis—pseudochondroplasia
    E. Coffee bean sign—caecal volvulus

25. **ROC (Receiver operating characteristic curve):**
    A. Is a graph of sensitivity versus specificity
    B. Is used to compare reporting of radiologists
    C. A diagonal line represents best results
    D. Accuracy is high when the curve follows the left hand border and then the top border of ROC space
    E. Increase in sensitivity is accompanied by decrease in specificity

26. **Contrast reactions:**
    A. Previous history of contrast reaction is usually elicited
    B. Adrenaline is given 1 mg, 1/1000 in 0.5 ml increments intravenously
    C. Hydrocortisone takes at least 30 minutes to show some effect
    D. 0.5 mg of ipratorium bromide is used for treatment of bronchospasm
    E. 10 mg of chlorpheniramine should be given as a fast bolus intravenously

27. **Contraindication for MRI using a 0.5 T magnet one month post-insertion:**
    A. Stainless steel coronary artery stent
    B. Titanium cerebral artery clip
    C. Sterilization clips on fallopian tube
    D. Cardiac pacemaker
    E. Spinal cord pain relief skin implant

28. **PET and SPECT scanning:**
    A. SPECT uses technetium and thallium isotopes
    B. Uses other substances than technetium
    C. Low glucose uptake is the basis of FDG scanning
    D. Utilizes anhilation of photons
    E. Absorbed dose is measured in MBq

29. **Parameters in MRI that will not decrease resolution or increase scanning time to improve image:**
    A. Alter FOV
    B. Phase encoding
    C. Shorter time to echo
    D. Longer repetition time
    E. Increasing matrix size

30. **Features of Down's syndrome in antenatal scan:**
    A. Short femur
    B. Polydactyly
    C. Increased nuchal translucency sign
    D. Pes cavus
    E. Pyelocalieactasis

ANSWERS

1. **A-F, B-F, C-T, D-F, E-F**
   Pain localised to fracture, less than 12 months old and pain refractory to medical management are common indications. Radiculopathy, cord compression, involvement of posterior aspect of vertebra with retropulsed fragment, sepsis and coagulopathy are contraindications.

2. **A-F, B-T, C-F, D-F, E-T**
   Cervical—anterolateral approach. Dorsal—transpedicular/peripedicular. Procedure is successful if superior and inferior end plate opacified and crosses midline. If cement enters paraspinous vein, procedure suspended till cement hardens. Methylmethacrylate cement is mixed with barium and tantalum/tungsten.

3. **A-T, B-T, C-T, D-F, E-T**
   Postbiopsy haematoma is a risk factor for spinal cord compression. Slight increased risk of fracture in weight-bearing bones, especially with large needles.

4. **A-T, B-T, C-T, D-T, E-F**

5. **A-T, B-F, C-F, D-T, E-F**
   Sclerotic lesions usually require trephine needles such as Ostycut Lytic lesions require small bore needles, including Chiba. Tru cut needles are also useful.

6. **A-T, B-F, C-T, D-T, E-T**
   Transpedicular approach usually does not cause CSF leak or tumour seeding, especially if the medial pedicular wall is intact. Biopsy through fracture mimics sarcoma due to tissue reparative processes.

7. **A-T, B-T, C-T, D-T, E-F**
   Pulmonary embolus results if cement enters paraspinous veins and then into IVC. Extension into epidural veins results in spinal stenosis and compression. Osteoporotic treatment should be continued.

8. **A-T, B -F, C-F, D-F, E-T**
   Nickel needles and carbon fiber needles are useful for MRI-guided biopsy. Carbon fibers reduce susceptibility artefact but visibility is low. Frequency encoding direction is placed parallel and phase encoding direction placed perpendicular to the needle track.

9. **A-T, B-T, C-T, D-F, E-T**
   von Hippel-Lindau disease is associated with cerebellar hemangio-
   blastomas and pheochromocytoma, along with renal cell
   carcinomas and cysts. Café au lait spots and small orbits due to
   dysplasia are features of neurofibromatosis.

10. **A-T, B-T, C-T, D-T, E-F**
    Thyroid carcinomas and neuromas are features of MEN syndrome.
    High-arched palate and arachnodactyly are features of Marfan's
    syndrome. Adriamycin is the common drug that is associated with
    cardiomyopathy.

11. **A-T, B-T, C-T, D-T, E-T**
    Short 4th metacarpal and depressed medial tibial condyle are
    features of Turner's syndrome. Peutz-Jeghers syndrome is
    associated with tumours of colon,small bowel, esophagus and
    pancreas. Acanthosis nigricans is a common dermatologic finding
    in neoplasms, especially carcinoma pancreas. Multiple enchon-
    dromas, Ollier's disease is associated with malignant transfor-
    mation, the most common being chondrosarcoma.

12. **A-T, B-T, C-F, D-T, E-T**
    Psychiatric disturbances, immunosuppression, infection, cataracts,
    diabetes, hypertension, fragile skin are other complications.

13. **A-T, B-T, C-T, D-F, E-F**

14. **A-T, B-T, C-F, D-F, E-T**
    Scleroderma is associated with alveolar carcinomas. Ankylosing
    spondylitis is an associated feature of inflammatory bowel
    diseases.

15. **A-T, B-F, C-F, D-T, E-T**

16. **A-T, B-F, C-F, D-T, E-F**

17. **A-T, B-T, C-T, D-F, E-T**
    Less than 10% of renal cell carcinomas calcify. Hydatid lung does
    not calcify due to constant respiratory movements of lungs.

18. **A-T, B-T, C-T, D-T, E-T**

19. **A-T, B-T, C-T, D-T, E-T**

20. **A-T, B-T, C-F, D-T, E-F**

21. **A-T, B-T, C-T, D-T, E-T**

22. **A-F, B-F, C-F, D-T, E-F**
    Celery stalk metaphysis which is irregular with vertical striations
    in seen in congenital rubella and osteopathia striata. Apple core
    is seen in annular constricting carcinoma of colon. Lemon sign and

Banana sign are ultrasound markers for open spina bifida. Hamburger sign is the normal appearance of facetal joint in CT and naked facet sign indicates facetal joint is dislocated.

23. **A-F, B-T, C-T, D-T, E-F**
Linguini sign indicates intracapsular rupture. Cottage loaf appearance is due to constriction of the liver passing through the ruptured diaphragm. Pancake vertebra is due to collapsed vertebra. Draping aorta sign is indicative of contained chronic leak.

24. **A-T, B-T, C-T, D-F, E-F**
Pop corn calcification is seen in pulmonary hamartoma and breast fibroadenomas. Licked candy stick appearance is seen in psoriasis, rheumatoid and leprosy. Champagne glass pelvis is seen in achondroplasia. Coffee bean sign is seen in sigmoid volvulus.

25. **A-F, B-T, C-F, D-T, E-T**
ROC curve is a plot of true positive rate against false positive rate for a binary classifier system. The closer the curve follow the left hand border and then the top border of the ROC space, the more accurate the test closer the curve comes to 45° diagonal less accurate the test. The area under the curve is a measure of text accuracy.

26. **A-F, B-F, C-F, D-F, E-F**
Previous history is usually not elicited.
Adrenaline IV route dose is 1/10000, 10 ml SC is 1/1000, 1 ml
Hydrocortisone takes at least 1-2 hours to take effect
Ipratorium bromide takes at least 30 min to act, so B2 agonists are used.
Chlorpheniramine is given slowly, diluted with 10 ml of blood.

27. **A-F, B-T, C-F, D-T, E-F**

28. **A-F, B-T, C-F, D-T, E-F**

29. **A-T, B-?, C-F, D-F, E-T**

30. **A-T, B-F, C-T, D-?, E-T**

13 *Miscellaneous*

1. Patellar malalignment:
A. Q angle is measured between the line joining anterior inferior iliac spine and the centre of patella and a line joining the centre of patella and tibial tuberosity
B. Q angle is best measured with the knee in 30 degrees flexion
C. Patellar tilt and trochlear groove depth are best assessed in lateral films
D. Spoiled gradient echo sequences are used for dynamic tracking of patella
E. Images are acquired at the level of trochlea to assess patellar tracking

2. Causes of resorption of the lateral end of clavicle:
A. Sarcoidosis   B. Trauma
C. Hyperparathyroidism   D. Cleidocranial dysostosis
E. Scleroderma

3. Congenital dislocation of hip:
A. More common in males
B. Associated with myelodysplasia
C. Acetabular angle is increased
D. Delayed ossification of femoral epiphysis
E. Alpha angle less than 50 degrees is always abnormal

4. Congenital dislocation of hip:
A. More common on the right side
B. Ultrasound is performed with 90 degree flexion of knee
C. Plain X-rays are the most useful in the neonatal period and ultrasound later on
D. It is good practice to delay the first ultrasound for 2 weeks after birth
E. Associated with femoral anteversion and hypertrophy of ligamentum teres

5. **Synovial osteochondromatosis:**
   A. Atleast 5 fragments should be present
   B. Due to metaplastic process
   C. Erosions and scalloping of bone is seen
   D. 11% recurrence rate
   E. Present in the first decade

6. **Hand injuries:**
   A. Scaphoid is most commonly fractured at the tubercle
   B. Triquetral fractures are best visualised in AP view with ulnar deviation
   C. Rotatory subluxation is best visualised in AP view with radial deviation
   D. In perilunate dislocation, the capitate is dislocated ventrally in relation to lunate
   E. Fracture of capitate is associated with fracture of scaphoid waist
   F. 75% of lunate dislocation is associated with scaphoid fractures

7. **Fibrous dysplasia:**
   A. High signal is seen in T2W images is a common feature
   B. Most common location is the spine
   C. No uptake is seen in bone scan
   D. 10% risk of malignancy in polyostotic form
   E. Not seen after epiphyseal fusion

8. **Fibrous dysplasia:**
   A. 70% of lesions are monostotic
   B. Inner table of skull is spared
   C. Sphenoid bone is most common skull bone involved
   D. Chondrosarcoma is the most common secondary malignancy
   E. Skull and facial bones are the commonest to undergo malignant transformation in polyostotic form

9. **Elbow injuries:**
   A. Dislocation is more common in the anterior than posterior direction
   B. The most common elbow injury in children is dislocation
   C. Radial head is the most common elbow fracture seen in adults
   D. Brachial artery injuries are more common than ulnar nerve injuries
   E. Periarticular calcification occurs in 20% of cases

10. **Musculoskeletal eponyms:**
    A. Wagon wheel fracture—Separation of proximal femoral epiphysis from rest of femur
    B. Snow boarder fracture—fracture of the calcaneum

C. Nursemaid elbow is olecranon fracture in child less than five years old
D. Nightstick fracture is usually associated with radial fracture
E. Jumper fracture—fracture of calcaneum

11. **Arthritis associated with nodules:**
    A. Neurofibromatosis
    B. Multicentric reticulohistiocytosis
    C. Amyloidosis
    D. Psoriasis
    E. Scleroderma

12. **Musculoskeletal ultrasound:**
    A. 90% sensitivity and specificity for diagnosis of supraspinatus tears
    B. Benign and malignant peripheral nerve sheath tumours can be differentiated easily
    C. Hyperechoic areas in tendon are always abnormal
    D. Cannot differentiate septic and aseptic effusions
    E. Normal subacromial space is seen as hypoechoic area

13. **Musculoskeletal ultrasound:**
    A. Xanthomatous deposits are hyperechoic within the tendons
    B. Tendon xanthomas are pathognomonic of familial hypercholesterolemia
    C. Plantar fascia is thickened if more than 4 mm
    D. Ankle effusions are best seen in the anterior tibiotalar joint
    E. Most of the lipomas are hyperechoic relative to subcutaneous fat

14. **Glomus tumours:**
    A. There is no nerve in a normal glomus body
    B. 75% are seen in hand
    C. Nail pain worse at night and relieved by tourniquet
    D. Majority are intraosseous
    E. High flow is seen in Doppler
    F. Lack of enhancement in MRI

15. **Musculoskeletal AIDS:**
    A. Tumours are the most common complication in AIDS
    B. Staphylococcus aureus is the most common cause of cellulitis
    C. Superficial cellulitis does not extend below the dermis
    D. Thickenning of deep fascia is in favour of necrotising fasciitis than cellulitis
    E. Intense rim enhancement is a feature of necrotizing fasciitis

16. **Musculoskeletal infections:**
    A. Ring enhancement is a feature of pyomyositis
    B. Bacillary angiomatosis is caused by Bartonella henselae
    C. Higher incidence of psoriatic arthritis in HIV
    D. Lymphoma is the most common tumour in HIV
    E. Kaposi's sarcoma shows uptake of Thallium 201 and no uptake in Gallium scanning

17. **Percutaneous vertebroplasty:**
    A. Cement leak is the most serious complication
    B. The cement has cytotoxic effect against tumour cells
    C. Cement is not used in tumours in non-weight bearing bones
    D. Prone position is useful for cervical and thoracic levels
    E. Leak into the disc results in increased risk of vertebral collapse

18. **The following are indications of vertebroplasty:**
    A. Spinal tumour with epidural extension
    B. Diffuse metastasis
    C. Osteoporotic fracture within four months of onset
    D. Painful acetabular tumours
    E. Multiple myeloma

19. **Sarcoidosis:**
    A. MRI cannot differentiate the tophi of gout and sarcoid nodules
    B. Large bone lesions enhance on contrast administration, in MRI
    C. Arthralgia is a feature of Löfgren's syndrome
    D. Polyarticular involvement is the most early type of arthropathy
    E. Bilateral umbilicated nodules are seen in the musculotendinous junction

20. **Causes of Erlenmeyer's flask deformity:**
    A. Thalassemia
    B. Osteopetrosis
    C. Niemann - Pick disease
    D. Lead poisoning
    E. Pyle's disease

21. **Areas showing persistently increased symmetrical bone scan uptake even with advancing age:**
    A. Sternal angle
    B. Sacral alae
    C. Medial end of clavicle
    D. Acromion process
    E. Distal femur

22. **Associations of fibrous dysplasia:**
    A. Acromegaly
    B. Hyperparathyroidism
    C. Hyperthyroidism
    D. Café au lait spots
    E. Elevated alkaline phosphatase
    F. Cushing's syndrome

23. **Causes of hyperuricemia:**
    A. Milk alkali syndrome
    B. Psoriasis
    C. Ethambutol
    D. Hypothyroidism
    E. Sarcoidosis
    F. Hyperparathyroidism

24. **Spinal fractures:**
    A. Tear drop fracture dislocation is due to flexion with axial compression
    B. Extension tear drop fracture is due to avulsion by anterior longitudinal ligament
    C. Wedging is more common posteriorly than anteriorly
    D. Hyperextension fracture dislocation produce bilateral interfacetal dislocation
    E. Hyperflexion sprain causes mild anterior subluxation of affected vertebra

25. **Haemophilia:**
    A. Pelvic mass is a clinical presentation
    B. Skeletal maturation is delayed
    C. Subarticular cystic lesion is seen
    D. Increased bone density is a common feature
    E. Joint space narrowing is very rapid
    F. Pseudotumours require urgent surgical evacuation of blood clot

26. **Synovial osteochondromatosis:**
    A. Affects the synovial lining within the joints only
    B. All the fragments are visualised
    C. Majority are polyarticular
    D. Distal interphalangeal joint is the most common joint affected
    E. Malignant transformation is seen in 10%

27. **Haemophilia:**
    A. The effusion in hemophilia has higher density than normal
    B. Presence of irregularity in the subchondral bone indicates development of septic arthritis

    C. Avascular necrosis is a salient feature in shoulder, hip and ankle

    D. Subperiosteal type is most common in the fibula

    E. Intraosseous form mimics giant cell tumour

28. **Spinal fractures:**
    A. Extension tear drop fracture is usually associated with spinal cord injury
    B. In bilateral facet dislocation, the anterior subluxation of vertebra is less than half of vertebral body diameter
    C. The articular facets of vertebra above, lie posterior to those below
    D. In unilateral facet dislocation, the spinous process faces the side of dislocation
    E. Bow-tie pattern in bilateral facet dislocation is seen below the level of dislocation

29. **Acetabular fractures:**
    A. Fractures of posterior wall are more common than anterior wall
    B. The most common acetabular injury is fracture involving both columns
    C. Anterior column fractures disrupt the ilioischial line
    D. Judet's views are obtained with the patient in posterior oblique position
    E. Spur sign is exclusively seen in both column fractures

30. **Wrist injuries:**
    A. Wrist dislocations are due to ulnar deviation of dorsiflexed wrist
    B. Disruption of proximal radiocarpal arc indicates perilunate dislocation
    C. In normal lateral view, the radius, lunate and hamate should be aligned
    D. In perilunate dislocation volar radiocarpal ligament is intact
    E. Wedge of pie appearance is seen in lunate dislocation
    F. Lunate dislocation is more common in the dorsal direction

31. **Hemodialysis is associated with:**
    A. Avascular necrosis
    B. Sacroiliitis
    C. Carpal tunnel syndrome
    D. Rupture of Achilles tendon
    E. Discitis

32. **Causes of high signal in T1 weighed images of synovium:**
    A. Pigmented villonodular synovitis
    B. Lipoma arborescens
    C. Still's disease
    D. Synovial osteochondromatosis
    E. Hemoarthrosis

33. **Fracture of coronoid process of ulna:**
    A. The site of common extensor origin
    B. Associated with anterior elbow dislocation
    C. More than 50% fracture is seen in Type 2 injury
    D. Brachialis inserts into ulnar tuberosity
    E. Heterotopic bone formation is seen in 40%
    F. Anterior fat pad is prominent

34. **Erosion of posterior aspect of calcaneum is seen in:**
    A. Gout
    B. Hyperparathyroidism
    C. Reiter's syndrome
    D. Acromegaly
    E. Scleroderma

35. **Progressive destructive shoulder arthropathy:**
    A. Most common in elderly females
    B. Basic calcium phosphate crystals are seen in the joint fluid
    C. Rotator cuff is torn
    D. 80% have blood tinged joint fluid
    E. Calcification is uncommon

36. **Ulnar subluxation at MCP joint without erosion occurs in:**
    A. Gout
    B. Jaccoud's arthritis
    C. SLE
    D. Psoriasis
    E. Rheumatoid arthritis

37. **Arthritis mutilans is caused by:**
    A. Leprosy
    B. Reiter's syndrome
    C. SLE
    D. Scleroderma
    E. Diabetes

ANSWERS

1. **A-F, B-T, C-T, D-T, E-T**

   Q angle is measured between the line joining anterior superior iliac spine and centre of patella and a line joining the entire of patella and tibial tuberosity. It is an indicator of valgus force exerted on patella with contraction of quadriceps mechanism. This is best measured in 30 degrees of knee flexion with patella located in the trochlea. A continuous 10 second exposure without table movement is essential in helical CT for assessing patellar tracking. Patellofemoral alignment is the static relationship between patella and trochlea in knee flexion. Tracking is dynamic alignment during knee motion.

2. **A-F, B-T, C-T, D-T, E-T**

   Rheumatoid arthritis, hyperparathyroidism, metastasis, multiple myeloma, cleidocranial dysostosis, pyknodysostosis, post-traumatic osteolysis, osteomyelitis are other causes.

3. **A-F, B-T, C-T, D-T, E-T**

   Congenital dislocation is 4-8 times more common in females, due to high levels of estrogen and relaxin at birth, which cause ligamentous laxity. It can teralogical, associated with myelodysplasia, arthrogryphosis and other neuromuscular disorders or it can be developmental in neurologically intact infants in the perinatal period. Normal acetabular angle is 28 degrees at birth and it progressively decreases due to modelling of acetabulum and femur. It is increased in dislocation. Normal alpha angle is more than 60 degrees, 50-60 degrees can be physiological, less than 50 degrees is always abnormal.

4. **A-F, B-T, C-F, D-T, E-T**

   More common on the left side (Because of the normal left occipitoanterior position in utero, the abduction of left hip is limited against maternal spine). In the first two weeks, any instability that is detected can be transient and it is useful to wait for 2 weeks. Ultrasound is useful in early stages, before the femoral head is ossified. X-rays are used after ossification. CT scan shows femoral and acetabular anteversion, hypertrophied ligamentum teres, fibrofatty hypertrophy of pulvinar and retraction of iliopsoas capsule.

5. **A-T, B-T, C-T, D-T, E-F**

   Other causes of calcified fragments are osteophytes, osteochondritis dissecans and trauma. More than 5 should be present for diagnosis. The disease is due to metaplasia of synovial lining. There are three stages. Synovial metaplasia without loose bodies, metaplasia with loose bodies and loose bodies without metaplasia. Erosions and scalloping are due to pressure of the fragements. Secondary osteoarthritis is a complication. Presents in 3-5th decade.

6. **A-F, B-F, C-F, D-F, E-T, F-F**
Scaphoid is most commonly fractured at the waist. Rotatory subluxation is best seen in AP view with ulnar deviation. Triquetral fractures are seen on the dorsal aspect in lateral film. Fracture of the capitate can be isolated, which is very rare or scaphocapitate type associated with scaphoid fractures. In perilunate dislocation, the carpal bones are dislocated dorsally 75% of perilunate dislocation is associated with scaphoid fractures, called the transcaphoid perilunate dislocation.

7. **A-F, B-F, C-F, D-F, E-F**
Fibrous dysplasia shows low to intermediate signal in both T1 and T2 due to fibrous component. High signal in T2 can be seen due to cartilage islands. High signal is also seen in children, more than subcutaneous fat. Bone scan shows increased uptake due to the vascularity of the lesion. Risk of malignancy is approximately 1%. Most common location is ribs. Craniofacial bones, proximal femur, tibia, pelvis are other locations. Usually seen in 5-15 group, but can be seen upto 70 years.

8. **A-T, B-T, C-F, D-F, E-F**
Majority of the lesions are monostotic. In the skull, the lesion always expands outwards, with thinning of the tables. Frontal bone is more commonly involved. Osteosarcoma, fibrosarcoma are more common than chondrosarcoma. Skull and facial bones undergo malignant transformation in monostotic form, whereas femur and pelvic bones are affected in polyostotic form.

9. **A-F, B-F, C-T, D-F, E-F**
Posterior dislocation is more common than anterior dislocation and is due to fall on fully extended abducted head. The most common elbow injury in children is supracondylar fracture. Radial head fracture is the most common elbow fracture in adults(30%) followed by olecranon fractures(20%) and coronoid fractures(10-15%). Transcondylar fractures are common in elderly patients with osteoporosis. Neurovascular injuries are seen in upto 20%, with ulnar nerve more commonly involved than brachial artery. Periarticular calcification is seen in 3-5% of cases. Other complications are nonunion, malunion, avascular necrosis, myositis ossificans, Volkmann's ischemic contracture, osteochondral defects and loose bodies.

10. **A-F, B-F, C-F, D-F, E-F**
    Wagon wheel fracture—separation of distal femoral epiphysis from rest of femur
    Snow boarder fracture—fracture of lateral process of talus
    Nursemaid elbow—subluxation of radial head in children less than five years
    Nightstick fracture is isolated fracture of mid third of ulna
    Jumper fracture—transverse fracture of upper third of sacrum.

11. **A-F, B-T, C-T, D-F, E-F**
    Sarcoidosis, gout, rheumatoid arthritis, osteoarthritis, pigmented villonodular synovitis are other causes of arthritis associated with nodules.

12. **A-T, B-F, C-F, D-F, E-F**
    Ultrasound has high sensitivity and specificity in diagnosis of supraspinatus tears. Hyperechoic areas in tendons can be seen due to anisotrophy. Septic effusions are echogenic with internal debri. Normal subacromial space is echogenic and is hypoechoic when there is fluid collection. Nerve sheath tumours are seen as hypo-echoic fusiform masses with or without acoustic enhancement, with entering and exiting nerves, but differentiation of benign and malignant is not easy.

13. **A-F, B-T, C-T, D-T, E-T**
    Xanthomas are bilateral and are pathognomonic of familial disease. The tendons are thickened and show focal hypoechoic masses. Normal plantar fascia is fibrillar and less than 4 mm. Ankle effusion gives the characteristic tear drop sign in anterior tibiotalar joint. Lipomas can also be hypoechoic or isoechoic.

14. **A-F, B-T, C-T, D-F, E-T, F-F**
    Normal glomus body has an afferent arteriole, an anastomotic vessel (Sucquet-Hoyer canal), collecting vein, capsular portion and nerves, which produce pain. Majority are seen in the soft tissue under the nail bed. Pressure erosion and thinning of bone can be seen. Doppler shows high flow and can detect tumours as small as 3 mm. MRI shows high signal in T2 and shows intense enhancement in T1 contrast enhanced images.

15. **A-F, B-T, C-F, D-T, E-F**
    Infections are the most common complication of AIDS. Staphylo-coccus aureus and Streptococcus pyogenes are the common causes of cellulitis. Superficial cellulitis does not extend below the superficial fascia. Deep cellulitis involves the deep fascia. Thickening of subcutaneous fat, thick superficial fascia, low signal

24. **A-T, B-T, C-F, D-T, E-F**
Flexion tear drop is seen in the anteroinferior aspect of vertebral body, associated with soft tissue swelling and interfacetal joint diastasis, making it unstable. It is associated with spinal cord injury. Extension tear drop fracture is seen in the anterioinferior portion of C2. This can be associated with hangman's fracture. Wedging is more common anteriorly. Hyperextension fracture dislocation is associated with impaction fractures of articular faces, with anterior displacement of vertebral body due to dislocation. The lateral column is disrupted in AP view and articular facets in lateral film. No bony abnormality is seen in hyperflexion sprain.

25. **A-T, B-F, C-T, D-F, E-F**
Arnold Hilgatner scale of hemophilia in knee: 0—no changes, 1— soft tissue swelling, 2—osteoporosis, overgrowth of epiphysis, 3—subchondral cysts, squaring of patella, widened intercondylar notch, 4—narrowed cartilage space, 5—joint contracture, loss of cartilage space, disorganised joint, gross epiphyseal enlargement. Abdominal mass can be seen due to bleeding into retroperitoneal space. Pseudotumours are seen in 2% and are very common in the pelvis. These are haematomas at site of muscular attachments and cause pressure erosion of adjacent bone. They are prominent in pelvis at site of iliopsoas and calf at site of gastrocnemius attachment. They are hypoechoic in ultrasound and have varying signal in MRI with hypointense hemosiderin rim. Treatment of hemophilia is enough for management.

26. **A-F, B-F, C-F, D-F, E-F**
Synovial osteochondromatosis is due to nodular proliferation of synovial lining of joints, tendon sheaths and bursae. It is usually monoarticular. Affects knee, hip, shoulder and elbow joint. Malignant transformation is uncommon and is usually chondro-sarcoma. Fragments are visualised only if they are ossified or calcified.

27. **A-T, B-F, C-T, D-T, E-T**
Tibiotalar slant(undergrowth of lateral side of tibial epiphysis), squaring of patella, widened intercondylar notch, widened trochlear notch, enlarged radial head are other deformities seen in hemophilia due to epiphyseal overgrowth. Avascular necrosis is caused in shoulder, hip and ankle due to compression of vasculature by intra-articular bleeding. Subchondral irregularity can be seen in haemophiliac arthropathy itself and does not indicate septic arthritis. High density effusion is due to iron and this is best seen in elbow. There are three forms, intraosseous,

subperiosteal and soft tissue. Intraosseous lesions are common in the femur, pelvic bones, tibia and small bones of hand. These are expansile and trabeculated and mimic primary bone neoplasms. Subperiosteal type is common in the fibula, produce periosteal reaction, cortical atrophy and soft tissue extension. Soft tissue lesions have fibrous capsule and indent the adjacent bone.

28. **A-F, B-F, C-F, D-T, E-F**
Extension tear drop is not associated with spinal cord injury, unlike flexion tear drop fracture. Bilateral facet dislocation—Anterior subluxation is more than half the vertebral body diameter, anterior dislocation of articular masses above, bilateral laminar fractures above the level. Unilateral facet dislocation—anterior subluxation less than half the vertebral body diameter, spinous processes above the dislocation rotated towards the side of dislocation, bow-tie (oblique) orientation of vertebra above dislocation, dislocated articular mass, increased distance between the posterior surface of articular mass and spinolaminar junction.

29. **A-T, B-T, C-F, D-T, E-T**
Anterior column fractures disrupt the iliopectineal line and posterior column fractures disrupt the ilioischial line. Judet's view is obtained in left posterior oblique and right posterior oblique positions with the X-ray beam entering at 45 degrees to the patient. Spur is a strut of bone which passes from the sacroiliac joint to the articular surface of acetabulum, which is disrupted exclusively in both column fractures.

30. **A-T, B-F, C-F, D-T, E-F, F-F**
In normal wrist the radius, lunate and capitate are in a straight line in lateral view. In AP view, the proximal radiocarpal row and distal intercarpal arcs should be smooth. Disruption of proximal arc—lunate dislocation, distal arc-perilunate dislocation. In perilunate dislocation, lunate maintains its alignment with distal radius, but the other carpal bones are dislocated. The scapholunate, lunocapitate and lunotriquetral ligaments are disrupted. Wedge of pie appearance is seen. In lunate dislocation, volar radiocarpal ligament is disrupted in addition to the other ligaments. Lunate dislocates volarly, but the remaining carpal bones maintain normal relationships.

31. **A-T, B-T, C-T, D-T, E-T**

32. **A-F, B-T, C-F, D-F, E-T**
PVNS shows low signal In both T1 and T2 due to hemosiderin. Synovial osteochondromatosis is hypo to isointense in T1 and can

have signal of cortical bone. T2 signal is high due to synovial hypertrophy or effusion.

33. **A-F, B-F, C-F, D-T, E-T, F-T**
The anterior bundle of medial collateral ligament inserts into the sublime tubercle and the brachialis inserts into the ulnar tuberosity. Regan's classification of coronoid process fractures, I—avulsion of tip, II—less than 50% fracture, III—fracture of more than 50%, A—absence of dislocation, B—dislocation. It is associated with posterior dislocation. Non-union, heterotopic bone formation, fibrous scar, recurrent subluxation loose bodies and synovitis are other complications

34. **A-T, B-T, C-T, D-F, E-F**
Psoriasis, erosive osteoarthritis, retrocalcaneal bursitis are other causes.

35. **A-T, B-T, C-T, D-T, E-F**
Progressive destructive shoulder arthropathy, also called Milwaukee shoulder is a crystal deposition disease, caused by basic calcium phosphate or hydroxyapatite crystals. These crystals produce prostaglandins, elastases and proteases which cause severe destruction of joint. Severe glenohumeral degeneration, humeral dislocation, chronic rotator cuff tear and calcific tendonitis are seen. It is common in elderly females. Joint fluid contains basic calcium phosphate crystals, particulate collagen, few leucocytes and collagenases and is blood tinged most of the times. CPPD deposition, overuse, renal failure, denervation and trauma are predisposing conditions. Can be seen in lateral tibiofemoral compartment of knee.

36. **A-F, B-T, C-T, D-F, E-F**
Jaccoud's arthritis is seen post rheumatic fever and causes non-deforming arthropathy.

37. **A-T, B-T, C-F, D-F, E-T**
Arthritis mutilans is a destructive arthritis with resorption of bone ends. RA, JRA, neurotrophic joints and psoriasis are other causes.

Bibliography

1. American Journal of Roentgenology, American Roentgen Ray Society.
2. Butler PF. Applied Radiological Anatomy, Cambridge University Press.
3. Clark KC, Naylor E, Roebuck EJ, Whitley AS, Swallow RA. Positioning in Radiography, Butterworth Heinemann.
4. Clinical Radiology, The Royal College of Radiologists, UK.
5. David Sutton. Textbook of Radiology and Imaging, 7th edn, Churchill Livingstone.
6. David W Stoller. Pocket Radiologist, Musculoskeletal Top 100 Diagnoses, Saunders.
7. Felix S Chew, Catherine Maldjian, Susan G Leffler. Musculoskeletal Imaging, A Teaching File, Lippincott Wiliams and Wilkins.
8. Grainger and Allison's Diagnostic Radiology, 4th edn, A Textbook of Medical Imaging, Churchill Livingstone Publishers.
9. Greenspan, Orthopaedic Radiology, A Practical Approach, 3rd edn, Lippincott, Williams and Wilkins.
10. Jamie Wier, Peter H Abrahams. Imaging Atlas of Human Anatomy, Mosby.
11. John AM Taylor, Donald Resnic. Skeletal Imaging, Atlas of the Spine and Extremities, Saunders.
12. Manalfe, Imaging of Spine and Spinal cord, Raven Press.
13. Manaster, et al. Musculoskeletal Imaging, The Requisites, Mosby.
14. Michael Brant Zawadzki, Pocket Radiologist, Spine Top 100 Diagnoses, Saunders.
15. Phoebe Kaplan. Musculoskeletal MRI, Saunders.
16. Radiographics Journal, Radiological Society of North America.
17. Radiographics, Radiological Society of North America.
18. Radiological Clinics of North America, Saunders.
19. Radiology, Radiological Society of North America.
20. Resnick, Diagnosis of Bone and Joint disorders, Saunders.
21. Rogers, Radiology of Skeletal Trauma, Churchill Livingstone.
22. Ryan S, McNichols. Anatomy for Diagnostic Imaging, Saunders.
23. Seminars in Roentgenology. Saunders.
24. Stephen Chapman, Richard Nakielny. A Guide to Radiological Procedures, Saunders.
25. Stephen Chapman, Richard Nakielny. AIDS Radiological Differential Diagnosis, Saunders.
26. Stoller. MRI in Orthopaedics and Sports Medicine, Lippincott Williams and Wilkins.
27. Theodore E Keats, Mark W Anderson. Atlas of Normal Roentgen Variants that may Stimulate Disease, Mosby.
28. Whitehouse GH, Worthington Brian S, Whitehouse Graham H, Worthington BS. Techniques in Diagnostic Imaging, Blackwell.
29. Wolfgang H Dahnert. Radiology Review Manual, 5th edn, Lippincott Williams and Wilkins.